Ad

"Joan Foust has written a must-rea͏d [...] to an aging loved one or parent. Read this book and learn from the best. I found it to be a delightful and insightful guide full of important and relevant information, with 'real-life' examples of 'what worked' and end results/successful solutions to assist on this journey."

— Lauren Simpson, RN, BSN
    Former President and CEO of Potomac Home Health and Potomac Home Support, Rockville, Maryland
    President of Simpson Nurse Consultants

"Joan writes with the same gentle voice as the caregiving practices she shares. Drawn into the real-life stories, I felt as though I was being accompanied by a wise mentor and encouraging guide. With each chapter, caregivers are equipped with fresh ideas that renew joy, restore hope, and instill confidence in life-giving relationships."

— Reverend Kirstin Tannas
    Pastor, Good Samaritan Lutheran Church, Solomons, Maryland

"In the post-Covid era, when quality care for our senior loved ones is ever more scarce, challenging, and expensive, Joan offers understanding, encouragement, and hope to us who take on the role of caregiver. Every one of the twelve chapters contains Joan's invaluable insights through real-life experience and stories. I pray that my loved ones will have read this book when it's my time to trust my health and independence to them as caregivers."

— Dr. Theodore Tsangaris, MD, MBA, FACS
    Vice President, Medical Affairs
    Chief Medical Officer and Program Director, Cancer Center at CalvertHealth Medical Center, Prince Frederick, Maryland

"Joan's book is amazing and I was touched by so many points. I loved the Try it Out segments—very useful and practical. I also loved the emphasis on being curious, which avoids the 'making assumptions' thing. And so much more—wow!"

— Dr. Jean Fleming, EdD, RN
    Former Executive Director of Calvert Hospice of Maryland

"I kept Joan and all her advice in my heart and mind as I spent the time by mother's side during her final days. I am so grateful for her sharing during our Business Impact Group meetings. Her words were my everyday guide."

— **Rick Amos**
Founder and leader of Business Impact Group, Maryland and Virginia
Mortgage Loan Officer at FitzGerald Financial Group, Maryland

"I rubbed shoulders with Joan Foust when she pioneered HomeLife as the managing partner/RN care manager in the late 1990s. She had a unique family-like dedication to her clients, aiming at finding such minute and major links to ensure they were well cared for. Joan's nursing background provided her the edge to manage clients' medical needs, giving them the comprehensive care they deserved."

— **Dr. Veena Alfred, PhD**
Certified Dementia Practitioner
Chief Executive Officer and Founder of AlfredHouse Eldercare, Inc.

"As a nurse practitioner and former family caregiver, I highly recommend this book for its practical tips and sage advice for the challenges of caregiving."

— **Nanette Lavoie-Vaughan, CGCP, APCNP-C, DNP**
Nurse Practitioner and healthcare consultant, educator, and author
National speaker on geriatric nursing and eldercare issues

Creative Caregiving Solutions

A Peaceful Approach
to Navigating Your Relationship
with Your Aging Loved One

Joan M. Foust, RN

HomeLife Press
Solomons, Maryland

Copyright © 2023 by Joan M. Foust
All rights reserved, including the right to reproduce this book or portions thereof in any form whatsoever without permission from the publisher, except as permitted by U.S. copyright law. To request permission, contact the publisher at www.JoanMFoust.com.
First paperback edition September 2023.

Contributing author and copy editor: Drew Drozynski
Developmental and copy editor: Elaine Klonicki
Front cover draft and proofreader: Jenni Hart
Cover and interior book design: Zach Wiggin
Front cover image: Richard de Ruijter at Unsplash.com
Dragonfly image: Rauno Tolonen at EasyDrawingGuides.com

Website: www.JoanMFoust.com

Facebook author page: www.facebook.com/CreativeCaregivingSolutions

The information provided in this book is for educational purposes only, and is not a substitute for professional medical advice for caregivers or their patients or loved ones. The advice offered represents opinions or judgments based on the author's professional and personal experience. Please consult a medical professional or healthcare provider if you require medical advice, a diagnosis, or treatment. The names of individuals in this book have been changed to protect their identities.

Library of Congress Control Number:
2023915944

ISBN: 979-8-9879564-0-3 (paperback)
ISBN: 979-8-9879564-1-0 (eBook)

Dedication

To my dear son Greg for always being
so supportive of me during your short life:
thank you for the beautiful signs you send
me now. The dragonfly, a symbol of growth
and transformation, is my favorite. It sits
with me on the porch sometimes
and encourages me to write.

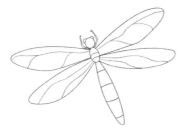

CONTENTS

PREFACE

Ever since I can remember, I wanted to be a nurse. My numerous hospital visits for asthma as a child and my surgery for a perforated appendix as a teenager may have influenced my determination since the nurses I encountered showed me such kindness and care.

After high school, I was offered a full scholarship to Abington Memorial Hospital School of Nursing near where I grew up. It was a three-year Registered Nurse (RN) diploma program that included classes at Penn State, Ogontz Campus, in Philadelphia, Pennsylvania. We had hands-on practice in every focus area in a 500-bed teaching hospital. The curriculum was structured to teach us the rationale behind our decisions, rather than just have us memorize what to do. We were required to demonstrate every procedure many times so that we would have a very high-quality skill set. While in school, I also worked on Saturdays as an aide at a nursing home which allowed me to learn even more about the basics of care for patients (while earning a bit of spending money).

My scholarship required one year of paid, full-time work at the hospital after graduation. I was a charge nurse overseeing a twenty-bed medical/surgical unit. It was demanding and fast paced, but I loved every moment of it. After that, I worked in a specialty eye and ear hospital, and then a plasma center.

When I switched to a long-term care center and began to work with aging adults, I found it extremely rewarding. It was so important to me to be allowed more one-on-one time with residents who were generally healthy but disabled due to age or some impairment. I was initially assigned to a "locked unit" for dementia residents (who tended to wander away if doors were able to be opened freely) and found that I was adept at working with residents with memory loss and confusion. Working with these patients would become my specialty in the coming years.

Over time, I worked in three different facilities in their memory loss units. Each of the facilities sent me for additional training on dementia care. Eventually, I became a nurse manager of thirty-eight residents at a memory loss center. Many difficulties and tricky situations arose as we provided care to the residents. When the situation became a struggle, such as when a resident refused to shower, I was called in to intervene. Together, the aides and I worked out peaceful ways to provide quality care for all the residents.

Although I was successful in these facilities, I always felt that having even more individual time with patients would be more rewarding than dividing my time among a large number of residents. When I was in nursing school, the rotation I liked best was being a visiting nurse, working with individual patients in their own homes. It was fascinating to me at the time and I had hoped to work in home health when I graduated. However, when I first applied, I was told I needed more experience. Initially I was crushed, but later realized that they were right—home care requires the ability to work independently (and bravely, at times), visiting many homes without easy access to other professionals.

After twenty years of nursing experience, I decided to try again and finally became a home care nurse. It was a very good fit. After three years, I was promoted to a supervisory role, and later became a manager of the supervisors. Finally, I was asked to be the director of professional services of the home care agency where I worked. Though it was a huge responsibility overseeing medical/surgical nursing, psychiatric nursing, physical therapy, occupational therapy, speech therapy, social work, and home care aide services, it was also an incredible experience that filled me with joy.

As director, I practiced really listening to staff and patient concerns and worked together with them to come up with solutions. I had developed my own style based on my value of peacefulness related to patient care. I found that I could encourage patients rather than force them, with better outcomes. This often took a bit more time to achieve, which was of course at a premium in home care being billed to insurance. Eventually my staff acknowledged that my nonconfrontational methods were more successful, but they still thought I was too optimistic about what could actually be accomplished within the constraints of the deadlines that were imposed on us. They joked that I must have been wearing rose-colored glasses to be so optimistic. I loved the job, but over time I found that my personal approach would be better utilized in situations where I could take more time with individual clients.

I began to feel that I wanted to use my philosophy of calm communication with patients to prove to myself that, in the long run, outcomes could be both more effective and more peaceful. As I grew more confident in this way of working, I started to consider establishing an independent practice. Just thinking about using my strategies out on my own gave me more and more energy.

Finally, in 1998, I made the decision to leave the agency. At our last meeting together, I gave each of my staff members a pair of rose-colored sunglasses in the hopes that they could now see what I saw—that these seemingly impossible things were possible with patience and determination.

I had discovered the geriatric care management movement (the overseeing of all aspects of home care for a patient), and decided this is where I would feel most useful. I started my own private pay care management company, which I called HomeLife Services, that same month.

For the first year or so, I worked on my own until I felt secure in care management, which required me to be skilled at more than just medical problems. I had to learn to handle many social issues for patients. It included medical/surgical care and teaching, as well as escorting patients to doctors and coordinating with everyone involved in a patient's care. I found new living arrangements for those who needed them, and helped ease the transition. I learned how to help patients think through their issues and how to work towards more comfortable and rewarding outcomes. I did mediation with patients' family members to help them better understand their loved ones' needs.

Eventually I had more referrals than I could handle alone, so I hired nurses and social workers with specific personality traits—especially patience, kindness, and determination—who shared my values. I was excited about sharing with them the communication methods I had developed with patients. I found that my staff had much to teach me as well, as they each brought special skills and viewpoints that benefited us all.

Our company provided professional care management for aging adults. As a private pay agency, we had more freedom and time to put our special philosophy into practice. Time for trust-building seemed essential to me, and I was proven correct in situation after situation as patients became more cooperative and the tension between family members and patients eased.

I managed the company for more than twenty years. I was able to continue to work directly with my own set of patients while overseeing my staff as they worked with theirs. It was challenging on many levels but also rewarding beyond belief. In addition to working with so many fascinating patients, one special part was the monthly session I had with my staff. I loved brainstorming solutions for the most difficult problems.

In these pages, I share many of the ideas from those sessions, where we discovered what worked (and what didn't) for all our patients.

My compassionate approach is one that can be learned by anyone who is interested in providing loving support to their family member or patient so they can be as independent, healthy, and happy in their environment as possible. I am thrilled that this book, which has been a longtime dream of mine, has finally come to fruition.

Best of luck to you,
Joan

FOREWORD

During our lives, we will probably give care, receive care, or both. Giving or receiving care ourselves is emotionally and physically taxing. We would all choose to live out our lives enjoying our independence, but this is usually not possible.

When the inevitable happens as we age or fall sick, friction among families can simmer or flare. The chronic nature of giving or receiving care for a family member can result in darts flying in both directions. It is a common family dynamic.

In the early 1980s, a few geriatric social workers, nurses, and gerontologists began to see the need for supporting these families by starting private care management practices. We were known as pioneers and frequently appeared in the media.

One of our responsibilities was to determine the quality of geriatric resources like nursing homes and home care. Then the families we served would not have to research on their own the most appropriate geriatric physician or retirement home for their loved one. We would be a one-stop shop.

It was in this vein that I met Joan Foust, who was working as an RN care manager at a local nursing home. I was impressed by how she interacted with residents and families. She had a natural warmth about her and showed a deep empathy for her residents, including many with memory impairments and psychiatric challenges.

With *Creative Caregiving Solutions*, Joan continues to give care, this time to her readers, by providing basic and essential coping methods for caregivers. Skills like listening, observing, and empathizing may sound elementary, but can be forgotten when caregivers face mounting frustrations associated with caregiving. Joan offers sound advice on polishing these skills and maintaining perspective. Further helpful are her insightful scenarios, in which Joan models these coping methods.

Inevitably, impatience, irritation, and other negative feelings will rear up all along the caregiving path. This book can be read and reread to keep one on a steady course with a professional guide for support.

Barbara Kane, LCSW-C
Founder, Aging Network Services
Psychotherapist
Co-author, *Coping With Your Difficult Older Parent*

INTRODUCTION

Caregiving for those who are aging or ill can be an emotionally taxing and physically difficult job. Still, many people choose to make it their life's work. They are special people indeed.

Often, however, the task falls into someone's lap as a newly required duty in an already busy life. Sometimes the caregiving role comes about gradually as parents, aunts, uncles, or siblings age and need more help. Other times a family member suddenly has a dramatic health event and needs both immediate and ongoing care.

When we reach adulthood, and as our parents and relatives start to age, we may begin to wonder what role we will have to take in their care. But even if we have a general sense that we will be called upon at some point, when it actually happens, it often feels like an unexpected journey. I understand. In addition to running my business, I was heavily involved in my own parents' care for many years.

Caregivers can find themselves dealing with medical, safety, and housing issues but also the emotional challenge of helping their family member to accept their new reality and to accept the necessary care from others. For many, navigating this emotional burden is more difficult than providing the care itself. Many decisions need to be made, sometimes quickly.

Whether it comes about gradually or suddenly, at some point it becomes clear that your loved one cannot manage on their own. When that time comes, one relative is typically designated as the primary person to manage their healthcare. This "family caregiver" is also the main contact person who talks with all family members to coordinate who will do what to fulfill the patient's needs. Most people don't have any training for this role. Often, they are simply the only one who is willing or available to do it. (In some cases, there is no family member to help, so the loved one has to rely on friends or paid caregivers.)

The role can be rewarding, but also exhausting and frustrating, particularly if it continues for many years. The difficulties are often exacerbated by complicated family dynamics. As the work increases and the challenges mount, caregivers begin to feel overwhelmed and even burned out.

None of us want to think of our loved ones as being a burden, but let's face it: people who need assistance with daily living are often not at their best. Sometimes they don't realize they need help, but even when they do, they can be resistant to it. I've heard many people describe their aging parents as "difficult," "stubborn," and "unwilling to do the things I know they need to do to keep themselves safe." Memory issues can compound the situation.

Sound familiar? If you're in this position, this book is for you.

It's also for you if you are a professional caregiver, especially one who is new to the field, and it can be useful for anyone in the medical field trying to encourage more patient compliance.

After having been a nurse for thirty years, I started my own business, HomeLife Services, to assist patients and families with their home health needs. *Geriatric care managers* like me are professional nurses or social workers or geriatric specialists who help aging adults work toward increased safety, improved health, and fulfillment in life. We help patients make decisions when they are unsure. We take them to doctors and coordinate their care. Mostly, we understand the life issues of the geriatric population and are adept at helping patients and their families consider all their options when it comes to living arrangements, transportation, and anything else that affects their quality of life.

Some of my patients have had physical disabilities or mental health issues, but for the most part I have worked with aging adults. I've always had great compassion for the family members who contacted me for help. I've been able to offer them hope, even from the first phone call. I knew from my experience that I could help turn things around with them and the person they were caring for.

The purpose of this book is to share my experiences so you can benefit from what I've learned over the course of my career. Hopefully these ideas will enable you to solve many problems, heal relationships, and will make caregiving much less frustrating for you.

Over the years I have developed my own approach for dealing with difficult situations and intractable problems in a way that is calm and solution-oriented, and resolves even longstanding issues. It is based on a list of principles and values that, taken together and applied over time, strengthen the connection between the caregiver and the patient. I have shared my method with the many nurses and social workers who have worked with me, but I've seen it work equally well for family caregivers like you.

In this book, I relate many stories about difficult problems my team and I faced with clients and the solutions that worked best for us. Because memory loss was my specialty, some of the stories are about dealing with that issue, but many of the tips I offer are applicable to all aging adults. My hope is that they will inspire you to work toward finding your own creative solutions for your loved one. You will figure out what works best for you.

Each chapter of the book focuses on a single principle, with several real-world examples to illustrate how I apply them with patients. Some of these principles will not be new to you, especially if you've done any caregiving with kids or even spouses who are ill. As you progress through the book you will learn to apply the principles using techniques that have been shown to work with seniors. The ideas build on each other, so the chapters are best read in order the first time (though feel free to peek ahead if a specific story title catches your eye). The "Key Takeaways" section provides you with a quick summary of the important points in each chapter, and the "Try It Out!" suggestions offer a way to start incorporating the concepts into your caregiving right away. As you read them, consider visualizing in your mind how you might apply a principle to your specific situation. If you're too tired or stressed at the moment to even think about trying something new, you can always come back to these suggestions when you are able.

It's important to understand that you will not be able to make all the changes suggested in the book in one go. After you read it through, you can think about which skills you already have, and those you will need to work on or refine. Choose one or two that speak to you, and start there. Go back and read those chapters again and consider ways to incorporate them into your caregiving role. Slowly add in new skills as you go along. If you're struggling to master a particular technique, it's okay to back off for now and try again later. All new forms of communication feel foreign to us at first, and it can take some time and practice before using them becomes a habit. Prioritizing skills and proceeding at your own pace will allow you to incorporate changes as you are ready. Note that if you are feeling particularly overloaded and overwhelmed right now with your caregiving responsibilities, you may want to turn straight to Chapter 12, which has suggestions for how to take care of yourself, and to the appendix titled "Hiring Home Care Providers" for tips on bringing in outside help.

My method will not make your role of caregiving easy. It's not a magic bullet. In fact, some of my patients' issues took months to resolve. But it will help. Remember, slowly but surely learning to use these new skills will lead you to more successful interactions. Conflicts can be resolved, and tensions can be eased over time.

I often hear from people that they can't believe I talked their parent into something when they were initially not cooperative. I feel I've had so much success with clients, even when others before me have tried, not so much because of *what* I do, but because of *how* I do it. I keep the principles I present in this book in mind as I approach each new situation, with the primary one being respect for the individual.

In the end, I hope you will feel like a better caregiver—more resilient and less stressed. As you develop the ability to solve the many problems inherent in the role you have taken on, you will make the lives of those you care for smoother, safer, and healthier.

I am thankful for each of you who has taken on the challenge of caregiving. Even if you don't always feel appreciated for the enormous effort you are putting into it, know that you are contributing to a better world for all of us.

Note: Since the book is primarily for family caregivers, in most cases I have chosen to use the words "loved one" or "family member" or "relative" rather than "patient" to reference the person you are caring for.

CHAPTER ONE

RESPECT

I've always been a peacemaker, and I learned over the course of my career that my specific gift is helping those who resist care to cooperate willingly. A lot of what I've done as a geriatric care manager is to teach family members a new way of relating with their loved ones that is more likely to be successful. Over time I have developed and refined my approach.

I found it so unbelievably helpful to truly value the patient, esteem them, and have affection for them, as well as to believe them. This level of personal respect is the foundational principle for the rest of my philosophy.

What do I mean by respect? It doesn't mean you have to agree with the person you care for. It means thinking of them as a whole person—as an individual. It means to honor their worldview, even if it is very different from yours. We all have unique preferences, perspectives, and paradigms. Those we care for are no different. If the person you are caring for doesn't think you respect them and their worldview, it will make the rest of the issues much more difficult, or impossible, to solve.

In some situations, admiration may come easily, and I hope this is the case for you. Unfortunately, in many situations, finding something to appreciate about a loved one who we feel is unlikable or unloving or resistant to care can feel like an impossible task. Sometimes a parent is dominant, which makes it harder for a son or daughter to help. Sometimes a son or daughter is dominant, and the parents just want to be heard.

I have seen many conflicts that are rooted in this issue of dominance. When one person decides they are unequivocally right, they no longer feel the need to listen to others or forge a common ground to solve problems. They may not even agree that there is a problem. Instead, they spend most of the time trying to convince the other person that they are right. Many times, there is no true right or wrong view of a specific problem, and what is really playing out in these situations is a power struggle between the individuals.

So how can you learn to respect someone who is being dominant or difficult? It helps to be able to let it go, honor your differences, and honor their wisdom. The following sections explain each of these three concepts in more detail.

Letting It Go

To me, finding respect in difficult situations requires learning to let things that provoke us to just be and to look beyond the surface to find the real person within who is suffering at the moment. Early in my career, I had to learn to let so many things go. To stop taking comments personally and look more deeply for what the patient was really trying to tell me. It's easier to reach a person if we can understand what is within them. This can be very hard to understand until we find what is triggering our own irritation with the person. Is it a memory of negative experiences from long ago? Sometimes it's not really their current behavior that is bothering us directly, but rather that it triggers frustrating memories, especially memories about how we were not permitted to behave similarly in our own past.

In my experience, many of these dominant and difficult behaviors are expressed when a patient is not feeling heard or validated in the first place. It's a vicious cycle, and one that tends to continue if we don't break the cycle by finding a way to appreciate them in some sense and listen to them.

It took practice for me to "look beyond" some years ago when I was helping my own mother. She was a beautiful, talented, gifted person who made this world a better place in so many ways. My challenge was to get past the disagreements that she and I had had when I was growing up. I had to let them just "be" in the past. As she grew older, she truly needed my help, especially since I am the nurse of the family. I will always love her, but I had to work hard to get past our differences. My early struggles with her actually taught me how to get along with people with very strong views, which in the end taught me to be a better care manager. For that I thank her.

Honoring Your Differences

One of the things that has helped me affirm and respect patients whose behavior is difficult is to focus on the fact that people are all different and have different ways they perceive the world. By honoring your differences, you can show the other person that you accept their viewpoint, even if you don't agree with it.

You may be familiar with the Myers-Briggs Type Indicator, which categorizes people into sixteen different "types" based on differences in the ways individuals prefer to use their perception and judgment. There are many other personality tests and interpersonal relationship quizzes that similarly define categories that people fit into. The key here is not the details of these systems, but what they all point to: there really are different ways that humans perceive and judge the world.

It is absolutely critical to recognize them as real, tangible differences! People often become argumentative when someone is coming to a very different conclusion than theirs based on the exact same information. One party will think the other party just "doesn't get it." We may decide that they simply must not know all of the information we know, because if they did, they would surely see it our way. But that is not the case. It's not just a matter of them not knowing what we know.

People truly do think differently. They organize differently. They process differently. They have different preferences. They judge things differently.

Everyone sets up their own internal systems for how they are going to interact with the world, and they are under absolutely no obligation to make their systems look anything like ours. By understanding that these differences are real—not just a misunderstanding or a lack of information—we can change our approach from trying to inform or convince to trying to listen and understand.

This fundamental shift in thinking is a core concept of this book. It will allow you to view frustrating situations differently and intentionally choose more thoughtful words which will, in turn, inspire a change in your loved one's level of cooperation.

Honoring Their Wisdom

One concept that helps me keep respect at the forefront is to focus on honoring the wisdom of seniors. Most have done quite well up to this point in life! Many have led amazing and consequential lives full of adventure and accomplishment. All of them know at least one thing we don't know, even if it is just what it was like to be a kid a very long time ago. They didn't get to the position they are in now by being told what to do all the time, so it helps to encourage rather than direct them.

We all deserve respect, and in offering it to those we care for, we can eventually earn their trust. This helps us to be able to solve problems with them, which is one of the goals of caregiving.

You may have a very different understanding of what "normal" means compared to someone who grew up a long time ago. Take personal hygiene, for example. In modern Western society, we generally take a daily shower. One hundred years ago, however, no one showered or bathed that frequently. People who are ninety-five years old did not grow up getting a shower every day, and many simply do not see it as necessary. Why would they?

People who were raised in different countries or different cultures can also have drastically different cultural norms from what you would consider "normal." An important aspect of respecting a patient's viewpoint is to work to figure out what their norms are and help them get close to those in their current circumstances.

If all a family member wants is one shower every few days and it is a huge ordeal to make a shower happen, there is no reason not to honor that request. The important part—the core thing we are trying to achieve—is cleanliness, not necessarily showering. It is critical to always consider the main goal of any activity, beyond the simple notion of "everyone does it that way."

There are many ways of achieving cleanliness. By looking at the core result you want, in this case cleanliness, you can find other potential solutions such as just washing up at the sink. If you only focus on the act you are trying to get someone to perform, and get stuck on that, you can miss other potential options and everyone ends up frustrated. I like to keep in mind what a patient's preferences are and see if most of them can be honored. I often find that I can achieve core goals while still honoring personal preferences.

The following stories illustrate my understanding of respect and how it can be applied in various real-world scenarios:

Tell Me How It Healed

On one of my home health visits I met an incredible senior gentleman named Jon, who had been an orthopedic surgeon. Unfortunately, Jon couldn't remember much anymore. His wife, Sherry, called me for help since she needed to leave the home at times. She said he would not stay with anyone. She also told me I wouldn't be able to have a conversation with him due to his memory issues and that he would panic if she left the room.

When I visited, I made sure to call him "Doctor" to show that I respected him and his knowledge. Rather than jump right into the issues at hand, I first wanted to demonstrate my esteem for him and build a level of trust and mutual understanding that would benefit us both. So, I engaged him further in his area of expertise:

I said to him, "I wish you were around when my granddaughter broke her arm. It seems to have healed strangely."

He asked, "Tell me how it healed."

I said, "It bends back too far at the elbow."

"How old is she?" he asked. I told him she was ten years old.

"Oh, she'll grow out of that," he offered.

Even though his short-term memory was quite limited, his long-term memory was apparently intact—at least regarding medical issues. He seemed to be proud to be able to help me (although I don't actually know if his statement was correct).

I told him that I was a nurse and always wanted to learn more about medicine. I pulled up a TED Talk on my phone about a medical discovery and he responded with intense listening. He had apparently been a master at many things in life, including wood carving, and he showed me some incredible carvings that were on his table. All this, from someone who was memory impaired! It might have been embarrassing to him to have only minimal access to all the words he needed to talk with me, but I completely understood him and he seemed calm.

What a gift to meet such an extraordinary man despite his current memory issues, and be able to help him relax. Sometimes we focus on a person's weaknesses—usually because those are the problems we feel we need to fix—but in so doing, we forget to draw on whatever strengths they still have. It was just amazing to hear him speak so clearly on medical issues when he normally struggled on a day-to-day basis to remember much of anything. His wife, Sherry, was so pleased!

This real mutual respect I developed with Jon through a simple conversation made it substantially easier to work with him in the future, even on difficult issues. Many people might see this interaction as a waste of valuable time. In reality, it was an investment to help him relax and trust me. This enabled him to accept his wife going out while I stayed with him.

I promise you that it is worth it to lay a foundation of respect in your relationship with your loved one.

She Shook Her Head "No"

One patient, Margaret, was in her late nineties and felt she wanted a break from any further medical care. She said she wanted no more hospitalizations, no tubes, no ventilation, and no more medical procedures. She specifically verbalized her choices and signed the request that she not be resuscitated.

When she suddenly had a massive stroke, the doctor at the hospital told the family she had only twenty-four hours to live. They took her back to her home and called in hospice. Many in her family thought they should at least give her an IV for fluids, or a tube feeding. They didn't think of those interventions in the same way as they would something like surgery or a ventilator. "Surely that wasn't what she meant," they said. This caused some dissension within the family, since others were arguing that she was quite clear on her instructions.

Even when patient instructions are clear, it is very difficult to wrap your head around the decision some make not to be helped anymore. No one wanted Margaret to be hungry or dehydrated, but she was unable to eat or drink by mouth. She was also unable to speak to confirm her earlier requests.

It's hard to accept a loved one's request when it conflicts with our own desires. This is quite a common reaction, and everyone needs time to consider their thoughts and emotions.

I arranged a group meeting with the hospice doctor and family to discuss options. The doctor said that an IV could cause too much fluid to build up in her lungs and she would be unable to process it normally. He also explained that their nearly one-hundred-year-old mother would not actually feel hungry, but rather would become weaker over time until she became unresponsive. With the family present, I went to speak with Margaret directly.

I asked her, "Is it okay if we give you fluids by IV?"

She shook her head to indicate "No" as a tear rolled down her cheek.

I'm glad she had enough energy in that moment to shake her head and truly clarify her desires for all. She made her wishes clear and they were subsequently followed. Her choices were honored as she had requested.

If she had not been able to shake her head, there could have been more arguments within the family. I hope this story illustrates that although honoring someone's wishes can be difficult, it is the right thing to do. Margaret passed away peacefully a few days later with her family by her side.

You may be angry at your loved one's decisions (how many arguments have you heard about who got left what in a will?), but it is important to respect that they are not your decisions to make. You are free to make your own choices about your life, and you can do things differently when you feel your end is near. But at the end of the day, our family members are the masters of their lives, and their decisions should be carried out to the extent possible. Isn't that what you would want?

"Yes, And" Instead of "Yes, But"

Once I was interviewing a woman, Dee, who had some memory loss. This was my first meeting with her, and we were in a circle with several family members. Dee said, "You know…I sleep very well at night."

I cheerily responded, "Oh that's helpful!" even though I was not sure if it was true. Patients often tend to minimize their issues, especially when meeting someone new. I followed up with a few questions about whether she got up to go to the bathroom. She stated again that, in fact, she sleeps quite well.

A family member interrupted at this point. "No, Mom. You get up three times a night!" The family member—understandably, I think—felt like the information being shared with the group needed to be accurate. Unfortunately, correcting someone with memory loss can remind them that they don't have a good memory and make them feel invalidated, or worse, stupid.

As a family member, it's important to remember that you can always make sure any medical provider has accurate information later, in private. In any group setting, it is best to just listen and let the loved one speak uncorrected.

As a caregiver, it is a good idea to inform family members, visitors, or other loved ones who may be tempted to make corrections that there will be a chance for further discussion afterward to make sure everyone has accurate information about the situation. Remind them that corrections in the moment are unnecessary. If it makes them more comfortable, family members can take notes about things said during group conversations that they feel should be corrected later.

If, for some reason, it is essential to make a correction, it's better to *add* to a story than to try to *correct* one. In improvisational comedy, there is a rule that you should always use "Yes, and" instead of "Yes, but." This allows each of the comedians to accept what someone has just said (the "yes") and add something to it (the "and"). Building on each other's contribution in this way allows you to create a flow of positive engagement in the scene. I think this is also a very good rule to follow for conversations with someone who may not be remembering everything correctly. Building a flow of positive engagement makes everyone involved feel good, and using "Yes, and" is a great technique for achieving it.

For example, the family member could have said, "It's good to hear that you can sleep, Mom, *and* I am glad it doesn't bother you that you have to get up several times to go to the bathroom."

Notice the difference? The exact same information is being conveyed, but it just feels nicer. It feels nonconfrontational. It is the kind of phrasing that allows everyone to stay comfortable and positive.

I am always careful to add to a patient's statements rather than correct them, especially when I take someone to the doctor's office. That way, the physician understands the situation more fully, but my patient still feels competent to speak about her own issues. You can always send a list of concerns to your loved one's doctor beforehand or use their health-care portal (if they have one) for further communication. Physicians are happy to answer follow-up questions with designated family members afterward as well.

———————

In this chapter I've offered several different ways to think about the concept of respect and some concrete examples of how to demonstrate it to your loved ones and those you care for. My goal in these stories is not to say there is one right way that is going to work perfectly every time, or that by pretending to show some regard you will get your way. Instead, I hope you can see how honestly affirming a loved one can change a relationship in a meaningful way, and that relationships founded on mutual regard just work better for both people.

I think we can all agree that it is easier to get things done if there is a good working relationship. Laying a foundation of respect first and treating people as people is really what we are all after. By seeing things through each other's eyes, we can find solutions that make sense to everyone. Through respect, many things are possible that otherwise would not be.

——————— **Key Takeaways** ———————

» Learn to let things that provoke you to "just be."
» Honor your loved one's wisdom and their point of view, even if it differs from yours.
» Focus on the core result you are trying to achieve, not on how it is accomplished.
» Make a human connection by focusing on their interests first.
» Follow your loved one's wishes whenever possible.
» Let them speak uncorrected in any group setting.

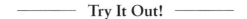

Try It Out!

Notice the difference when you add to your loved one's comments using "Yes, and" rather than correcting them. How does it change things?

CHAPTER TWO

LISTEN

Communication is a key tool for problem-solving, and the most important part of effective communication is listening. In addition to respect, active listening is a key tool in your solving-difficult-problems toolkit. In my experience, so many problems can literally dissolve when people take the time to listen to each other and fully understand what the other person is trying to say. Problems that do not resolve outright become remarkably easier to solve.

The opposite is true as well—if we don't listen carefully, we can create problems that would not have otherwise existed. Miscommunication is a major source of tension in relationships.

I learned the importance of listening to patients while I was just beginning my nursing program. I was asked to go around one of the units, check to make sure everyone received their breakfast, and see if they needed anything else at the moment.

One patient asked me if I would please go get him a donut. He said that he had already asked a few times. Trying to respond as quickly as possible, I immediately called down to the kitchen and had them send up a donut for him on a plate. When I took it to him, he said, "Oh. No... I was talking about an inflatable donut cushion to sit on. Didn't you know that I had hemorrhoid surgery?"

How frustrating for him and embarrassing for me! That was the moment I realized how easy it is to make an assumption about what someone is talking about. I heard his words, but I didn't really *understand* him. It's all too easy to hear something and assume you know what someone meant by it.

Listening works better when it's an active process. First you hear their words, then you confirm your understanding. From that day forward, I learned to confirm what I thought I heard. Oh, how I wished I had known that first time to say, "Sure, I can get you a donut. What kind would you like?"

There is almost no greater gift we can give to those in our care than to listen to them intently. It not only makes them feel heard and cared for, but it also helps us to learn what motivates them and what they are really asking for.

There are several techniques that can be used to gather more information to avoid miscommunications. They allow you to not only *hear* what is being said, but to *understand* the message being communicated.

Using Active Listening

Active listening is a term coined by psychologists Carl Rogers and Richard Farson in a paper they wrote in 1957, which became a book by the same name. The technique they described, which they sometimes called "sensitive listening," involves trying to see the world from the speaker's point of view. According to them, in addition to not allowing yourself to be distracted when listening, it's important to show the other party that you are staying focused on them by nodding your head and refraining from interrupting.

People usually like to tell us what life is like for them, and if we tune into what it feels like to them first, we are more likely to truly hear them. If we discount their feelings or jump to another topic, it can cut off the other person and make them feel less valued. Sometimes during conversations, we are hearing the words while thinking about what we want to say next, but waiting for someone to finish speaking is not the same as listening to what they are saying. Listening to what they feel they need or want is priceless. We can begin to comment at the appropriate time, but in a way that shows we really understand what they have told us.

Instead of thinking about what to say next, focus on how you will respond to clarify what you think you are hearing. You can show people that you care about what they are saying by restating their comments using different words to see if they agree with your summary. Asking follow-up questions can also demonstrate your interest and clarify your understanding. By being inquisitive and listening intently, you can begin to understand what is behind their behaviors or reactions and what motivates them in life. Gathering information in this way also demonstrates your respect for them—they can see that you care about what they think and say.

There is kind of an art to forming questions and repeating back what you have heard in a way that doesn't sound silly. For example, if someone says, "I go to the store every Friday," it is easy to make a lot of assumptions about what this might mean. It would be a bit awkward to respond, "I'm hearing you say you go to the store every Friday, is that right?" This doesn't allow you to gain any more information. Try asking something more specific, for example: "Oh, do you go to the mall?" They might respond, "No, that's when my husband drives me to buy our food for the week," and now you have gotten clarification on their meaning.

As another example, if someone reports that they haven't eaten breakfast, there could be several reasons why. Perhaps they normally eat breakfast, but they weren't hungry this particular morning. Or they don't normally eat breakfast at all. Or a new medication is making their stomach upset. To clarify, I might say, "Oh, so you're not a morning eater?" If they respond, "No, I've never really eaten breakfast," then I've gained some insight about their eating habits. If they respond, "I normally am, but I'm feeling nauseous today," then there might be a more significant issue to investigate. Over time, asking questions and restating what you are hearing to improve your understanding gets much easier.

For your loved one, the frustrating feeling that they are not being heard can rapidly dissolve as soon as you clarify what they are telling you. It usually takes just a few more minutes of your time, but because it can ease tensions so quickly, it can feel like a nearly miraculous moment. There will still be problems to solve. But easing tensions is no small feat, and all you have to do is listen intently and try to explain back to them what you heard until everyone is on the same page.

Active listening is a simple and remarkably effective tool to have in your toolkit. Consistently checking back to make sure we understand our loved ones, and responding carefully using words and phrases that are more likely to be effective, results in vastly better outcomes. Since active listening provides more information than regular listening, and builds more positive relationships, it is highly useful for helping people move toward change.

Using Motivational Interviewing

In addition to letting someone know you are genuinely interested in them, listening is also the best way to figure out someone's thoughts about an issue. It should be obvious to us that if you want to motivate someone, you should learn what moves them toward action! Unfortunately, this step is often missed, and as a result, caregivers often try to coerce or force something to happen instead of motivating the patient or loved one to come to a decision of their own accord. Studies have shown that this practice actually has the opposite effect—that when someone tells us what to do, our brains are actually wired to resist and do the opposite instead! This need to push back when we see our choices as being limited by someone else is referred to by psychologists as *reactance*.

Think of this in your own situation. Have you ever thought something like "My parents need to move into assisted living for their safety. They are being so stubborn about it." It may seem quite reasonable to have this kind of thought, and many of the families I have helped started by thinking this way. But a much more helpful thought is "How can I help my parents *want* to move into assisted living? What is motivating them to want to stay in their house?" See the difference?

In my career I have seen many problems that stem from a lack of understanding about why someone is doing what they are doing. What motivates their behavior?

It's critical to listen attentively to learn a person's rationale for doing things a certain way. The style of communication I am describing, also known as *motivational interviewing*, was originally documented by William R. Miller and Stephen Rollnick in the 1980s as a way to aid people with substance abuse disorders. Their book *Motivational Interviewing* is worth a read if you have the time to delve into this topic further. They provide detailed strategies for listening specifically to understand someone's motivations. When I started using this communication style, I had not yet heard of the concept, but noticed that I naturally used it to achieve good results.

The technique works especially well for the times when someone is resisting care and you don't understand why. Unfortunately, asking, "Why are you resisting?" is unlikely to get you very far. Instead, become curious about it. I often say, "I wonder what made that happen?" They may answer with something like "I think I was afraid." We can then explore further, using our curiosity as a guide: "I wonder what that fear is all about?" It is important to be continuously curious, not just superficially curious. Many people will ask the first question, but when they hear that the person is afraid, they will say something like "You don't need to be afraid of that." While this may seem reassuring, it is actually discounting their feelings. I know I heard that response many times in my early life when I expressed fear, and it made me feel dismissed instead of motivating me.

It's also important to ask just one question at a time and to wait patiently for the response. Aging adults and those who aren't feeling well often comprehend at a slower pace and can only think through one concept at a time. Give them the time they need to formulate their answer.

Too often, we come in with our thoughts about what is right for another person, but they have their own ideas, and we should respect that. It's up to us to use our communication tools to elicit these ideas from them.

Using "What" Instead of "Why"

Another helpful technique I learned in school was to use the word "what" instead of "why" when asking questions, as patients often feel defensive when asked a "why" question. I believe this is because "why" triggers a need for people to explain themselves. Watch the difference in a person's reaction when you use the word "what" to formulate questions. "What is the cause of that?" not "Why did you do it that way?"

Accusatory tones are often answered with the unhelpful response "I don't know." "I wonder what made that happen?" tends to draw out more informative answers. If I ask how they slept and they say "Terrible," I may be tempted to ask "Why?" but they may just say, "I don't know." If instead I ask, "I wonder what made that happen?" the response is usually more concrete and helpful, like "I think it was my back pain" or "My mattress is uncomfortable."

Using "why" can also feel like the person is the one who is supposed to have all the answers, which implies that they are in charge of solving these problems themselves. Many times, their response in this scenario will be to stop talking about problems they don't have a solution for, which is the opposite of what we want. If instead we ask, "What happened there?" it feels like we are engaged in problem-solving *with* them. Now the two of us can work together to identify possible issues and think of solutions together. Importantly, this doesn't mean that the problem is now *yours* to solve on your own either.

For example, if a family member says they didn't sleep well and you ask what happened, if they say "My mattress is uncomfortable," that does not mean you should run out and buy a new mattress. It means you have identified a possible problem together, and you can work to solve it together. My next line of questioning would continue the curiosity: "I wonder what it would be like if you had a new mattress or a memory foam topper?" Letting them give input into solutions is another key piece of the puzzle here, and it is also part of active listening and working to understand their deepest motivations.

Asking Low-Pressure Questions

Often as we age, we lose a bit of quickness in our thinking. Part of being a good active listener includes giving someone enough time and space to answer a question. By changing how we word things, we can grant our loved ones this time and space to process what we are offering without pressure from our side.

As an example, perhaps I think it would be a good idea for a patient to have someone cook for them rather than trying to handle it themselves. Of course, I could just ask, "Would you be okay if I got someone to come and cook for you regularly?" There is nothing wrong with this question *per se*, but in practice it can make it seem like you want a final answer right at that moment. In my experience, that final answer is more likely to be something like "No, I can cook for myself." People do not usually want to change their current situation since it is what they're comfortable with (even if what you are proposing seems to you like it would be more convenient). They may also feel that they are losing some independence if they make a decision like this, and losing independence is scary.

I have seen families ask questions like the one in the previous paragraph even when they already knew for sure their parent wasn't currently able to prepare a meal. They think that since they're going to get a cook anyway, they should at least ask their parent for permission. Unfortunately, this sets up an immediate argument if the parent says "No!" What is the next thing you would say after a parent says they can prepare their own food? "No, Mom, you know you can't cook for yourself right now." That sure sounds like the beginning of an argument to me. So how can we avoid this common trap?

One of the best ways I have found to ask questions without seeming like I'm trying to pressure someone is to *wonder about it out loud*. If I say, "I am trying to imagine what it would be like for you to have some-one cook your meals while you recover," it totally changes the kind of responses I receive. This phrasing drastically reduces pressure (they don't have to answer at all if they don't want to), gives them time to think, and directs them to genuinely consider what it might be like (instead of whatever knee-jerk reaction they would have if pressured). Plus, by asking their opinion and valuing their response, you are actually giving them more agency and independence, rather than making them feel like you are taking it away. As with all of these techniques, this will not au-tomatically make people do what you want. However, it will give them time to think it over without needing to give a direct answer immediate-ly. Remember, if you ask for a final answer right away about a potential change, the automatic answer is almost always to keep things as they are now, even if the change seems beneficial.

Allowing time for others to tell their story or letting them speak their mind can give them a feeling of closeness. Once you have taken the time to really listen and get everyone on the same page, it is tempting to start offering advice and guidance based on this newfound mutual understand-ing. However, if you follow their story with lots of advice, they often are not ready for it yet. Give them time to become comfortable with the new bond you share before trying to guide them. When you do feel the need to provide advice, try wondering about it out loud instead.

Whenever possible, we should utilize the information we get from our loved ones so they can see that it meant something. You don't want to just pay lip service by asking them what they'd like and then doing what-ever you want. You're trying to create opportunities for them to do what they'd like in a way that will make everyone's lives easier.

Listening to Those with Memory Issues

Listening can be a challenge when dealing with someone who can't re-member. It is tempting to discount things that they have said on one day if they completely forget about them by the next day. Does it really mat-ter what they said yesterday if they can't repeat it today? I think it does.

I have a special place in my heart for people with memory issues. It is my belief that when someone with impaired memory tells you something, even if you know they probably won't remember it tomorrow, you should listen in the moment anyway. If you can tell they understand, and they give you answers when you ask questions, that's how they're really feeling right then.

As caregivers, we can help remember things for them. They might not remember today what they said yesterday, but you can, and you can make sure to follow their wishes. Many people know something at the moment, even if it's fleeting. You can usually tell when someone "gets" something, and it would be a shame to discount that just because they have a memory loss issue. Their feelings are still valid even if they can't repeat the sentiment later.

Listening to Those Who Struggle to Communicate

Some people are capable of expressing themselves at times even though they do not initiate without prompting. They may talk if you make things simple enough. Try asking yes or no questions. It might not be obvious that someone is willing to give input so look for a time of day when they're most alert and aware.

For example, one of my patients was generally confused, and his social worker said it wasn't worth asking him about his wishes. With his doctor there, I got down to the level of his wheelchair and looked right into his eyes and asked him a question about future hospitalizations. The social worker was surprised that he responded to me. He said, "I want whatever will keep me alive the longest to stay with my wife." The doctor interpreted that to mean that he was okay being sent to the hospital for IV meds when he got infections.

My feeling is that you should never ignore someone's input—even small inputs matter, and it's always worth it to try. It's important to show other family members and/or their doctor what you are witnessing so they understand that the person at times still has the ability to respond. It can settle many questions, especially when there is a difference of opinion between family members. It's so worth trying to approach people when they are alert to see what they are thinking.

Because it helps so much to smooth things over, it's worth your time to always be on the lookout for assumptions and potential misunderstandings and to clarify things, especially when you seem to be disagreeing or there are tense feelings. It can really help bring calm and ease to a situation. When a person finally feels heard after a long period of feeling powerless, they can breathe a sigh of relief.

The stories that follow demonstrate how you can prevent misunderstandings with your loved ones by being a careful and caring listener:

He Loves to Drive

In addition to listening to a patient or loved one attentively, asking follow-up questions, and reiterating what the individual has said to ensure there is no miscommunication, it is important to also verify the information you are receiving from other sources. For example, when one gentleman I worked with, Arthur, was informed by his physician that it was no longer safe for him to drive, his wife, Maryanne, became upset. She pulled me aside and said, "Don't take driving away from him. He loves to drive. It's one of the most important things to him."

Later, when I was speaking with Arthur alone, I mentioned that I heard he loves to drive. I told him that I also love to drive, thinking we could discuss our mutual enjoyment of the activity, and maybe probe a bit to see how he might be taking the news. Then he said something unexpected: "No, I don't really care if I never drive again. I just always have to drive Maryanne around because she can't do it."

"So," I wondered aloud, "I wonder what it would be like for you to have a driver?"

"Well, who would do that for us?" he asked, intrigued.

It turned out his biggest concern was that he didn't want to take taxis everywhere. When I told him that we could find a regular driver who could pick them up and take them wherever they needed to go, he agreed. I began to look for a driver that very evening, searching the internet for "senior transportation" options in their area. Once I had found a reliable and trustworthy person, I took the time to sit down with Maryanne and explain that although Arthur has always liked driving in the past, he has been more tired lately and would like to try a driver for a while. She agreed to the plan as long as Arthur agreed. (Notice how I was very careful not to negate her original report to me on his love of driving?)

This story has a few elements that are worth thinking about. First, listen attentively, but always verify statements that you are hearing. Sometimes things can be seen very differently by different people in a situation, even if they think that they are all on the same page. Second, I "wondered" my idea out loud again. As I mentioned previously, this can be a powerful tool and often leads toward solutions without anyone feeling coerced or pressured. There are other techniques I employed in this situation—shrinking the decision by limiting it to a trial run and moving quickly once there is consensus—that I will explain in detail in later chapters.

My Daughter Is Coming This Weekend

It can be really tricky not to jump to conclusions when someone makes a statement. Our brains just seem to want to fill in the details for us from our own knowledge and experiences. Fighting this urge does not always come naturally, but once you have seen enough examples of how misunderstandings can happen, you start feeling more comfortable asking follow-up questions. I hope these examples can help you see that it is always good to seek a deeper understanding instead of assuming you know.

On a Friday afternoon one of my patients, Pam, said, "Oh, my daughter is coming this weekend." My first thought was to say, "Oh good!" but instead I paused for a moment, realized I didn't know how she felt about her daughter visiting, and asked, "What is that going to be like for you?" She replied, "Well, I can't stand when she comes because she smokes, moves my things around, and bosses me around the whole time." Since I enjoy spending time with my own daughter, it would have been easy for me to say "Oh, won't that be fun!" instead of figuring out how it felt to her. Instead, I showed her that I respected her as a separate person with her own thoughts and feelings, and was able to more fully listen to her and come to a better understanding of her situation.

When you hear new statements of any kind, it can be helpful to take a moment to pause and think about how you best want to respond before saying anything. The point is that you can't always accurately guess someone's thoughts, and it's good to remember that we don't know exactly what they are thinking.

Often, it is our first instinct to assume we understand, but if you can reflect for a moment, you can give yourself time to figure out whether there is anything missing from your understanding. I find it really helps me process statements more deeply than I normally would to avoid jumping to any conclusions. As you navigate conversations with your loved ones, try inserting these pauses to see whether you can think of questions to deepen your understanding of what they are really thinking.

I Can't Breathe

Once I was visiting a long-term care facility and as I was ready to leave, I noticed the staff standing around a resident who had just arrived for admission. Alice, who was in a wheelchair, had apparently just been dropped off by her son. Almost immediately, she started screaming and crying and saying over and over, "I can't breathe!" She got louder and louder. It's possible the son left because he expected her reaction and didn't have the capacity to handle it, but that's just a guess, because I didn't actually witness the drop-off. There were three staff members standing around her wheelchair trying very hard to calm her, but the screaming just got worse.

The staff looked at her and said, "It's all going to be okay, let's get you to your room." Though I was not a staff member, I felt compelled to intervene. I went over and bent down on one knee and said to the new resident, "You can't breathe?" She looked at me and said more calmly, "I can't breathe where there is carpet." I said, "Oh! I can take you outside away from carpets for a moment if you would like." With staff permission, I wheeled her outside on a side patio and talked with her.

"It's terrible that my son is putting me here," she said.

I sat next to her. "I don't know how all of this is going to work," I said, "but I understand that you need to be comfortable. There are no carpets in the resident rooms, so I could wheel you quickly to your room and get you a drink."

After a few minutes, she agreed and I took her to her new room and asked a social worker to follow up with her. She seemed to need to know that someone heard her concerns. The carpet might have actually bothered her, but she was also upset about her son's decision to admit her there. Her strong emotions about it were more than she could handle so she "lost it" when she first arrived.

One can make all kinds of assumptions—that it's a panic attack, or that she needs to just relax, or she needs to be medicated—but getting down to her eye level and letting her know she was heard de-escalated the situation. Just being calm, making eye contact with a person, and truly listening can help in so many scenarios. This situation went from highly emotional to calmer to solvable because I took the time to listen and show concern.

You Don't Know Me, But...

This chapter is mainly about us developing active listening skills, but I feel it's important to point out that patients are also always listening to us. They tune in to phone conversations to see if you bring up anything that you have not yet shared with them. This is true even if they're hard of hearing or nonresponsive. They can listen and absorb information even when they are asleep or comatose! We need to be aware of this when a patient is present and respect them by conversing accordingly.

Once I took care of a patient named Martha in the ICU who was comatose. As I cared for her, I talked and talked with her as I had been taught to do. After her recovery and return to another hospital unit, I visited her there and said, "You don't know me but..." She immediately interrupted and said that she knew my voice, even though she had been comatose when she heard it. I was so amazed. That experience taught me to recognize that hearing can remain functional during a comatose state. I learned this in nursing school but it wasn't until I saw it with my own eyes that it really stuck with me.

Sometimes family around the bedside discuss important issues while their loved one is sleeping or comatose. Hospice patients especially will listen in if we start to discuss what we will do after they pass. It helps to arrange another time or place to discuss issues of recovery or death when your family member is awake and communicating. Whether they are asleep or comatose, I can't stress enough the importance of speaking only about topics that you are comfortable having them hear as well.

––––––––––

The above examples show that focusing intently on a person's input promotes better understanding and allows our loved ones to feel calmer because they are feeling heard. It also allows us to better respond to them in a way that makes them feel understood. We all want someone to hear our situation and care about how we feel, so I try to give that to patients as much as possible. The feeling will be better all around.

Focusing on the motivation of others allows us to come up with ideas that will work better for our family members. Clarifying the meaning of their words decreases stress for all involved. The suggestions in this chapter are not always easy to carry out, but are certainly worth striving for.

——————— **Key Takeaways** ———————

» When our loved ones feel we are really listening, it makes them feel close to us.
» Allow time for people to tell their story.
» Show interest and restate what your family member has said to confirm your understanding.
» Ask low-pressure questions to determine their motivation.
» Use "what" instead of "why" questions to avoid triggering defensiveness.
» Instead of making suggestions, try wondering out loud.
» Take time to verify rather than assume.
» When someone is upset, get down to their eye level, speak calmly, and listen to them.
» Know that aging or ill loved ones are always listening even when you are unaware of it.

——————— **Try It Out!** ———————

Listen to how often you use the word "Why"
and try to change it to a "What" question.
Do you notice a better response?

CHAPTER THREE

OBSERVE

So far, I have covered respecting and listening to the people we care for in order to help them feel comfortable with our conversations. What we observe about their health, mood, environment, and communication style is just as valuable. We can glean so much by looking closely at all aspects of their life in order to ascertain their current needs and figure out what motivates them. The best way to ensure we are getting their input on their care is by both asking and observing.

As humans, each of us naturally observes one another and our world all the time. You may be surprised to hear, though, that what we actually take in can be vastly different. Some of us only see the big picture and others notice tiny details. (Both are important, for different reasons.) In addition, some people are naturally more adept at understanding and interpreting what they notice. But we can all improve our own skills with practice.

As you learned in the last chapter, listening is one way of gathering information. Observing provides us with another way to add to our knowledge of a person's needs. The reason it's so important is that physical and environmental issues can affect your loved one's moods, the way they communicate with you, and the degree to which they cooperate. If you can identify the issues that are making them uncomfortable or worried and help resolve them, it can often make the person feel better, which can make them more receptive. As you will see, working toward paying better attention to everything that affects the person you are caring for is well worth the effort it takes.

Nonverbal communication—communication that occurs without words—involves eye contact, facial expressions, gestures, postures, and body language. Looking closely at these can give us clues as to what someone is feeling, and help us be more in tune to how they might react to our suggestions. In this way, nonverbal clues can help strengthen our interpersonal relationships, which are so important when we are providing care.

Preparing Yourself

In our caregiving role, it is important to let go of our own concerns and concentrate solely on our patient or loved one so we can pay full attention to observing. If we appear to be stressed or rushed, or come off as too authoritative, they will pick up on it and the interaction will be strained from the outset. Even if we say all the right words, our body language may reveal that we're not really present.

Our self-talk is always rambling on, but we can put that aside for a little while for the sake of our loved one. Before I go into a house or room to meet a patient, I stop for a minute to remind myself to let go of any worries or anxieties or concerns I have in my own life. It helps me to take a breath and visualize the attitude I want to bring to the visit. I want to be happy and upbeat, so I put a smile on my face. Most of all I want them to feel that I am fully present with them.

I found this hard to do when I first started working in home health but got better at it over time. It is actually a relief at times to be distracted from our own issues.

At the same time, when you enter a loved one's room or home, it can help to make a mental note of what you observe and how it is affecting you. What do you concentrate on when you walk into a family member's environment? Are you attentive to their mood? What causes you to have positive or negative reactions? In my experience, patients really seem to appreciate when we look directly at them and appear interested in what's going on with them. It starts the interaction off on the right foot.

As we arrive for a visit with our family member, we can notice their demeanor and behavior to determine what means the most to them. What are they trying to express to us, even if they aren't communicating it verbally? Are we looking at them with an observant eye to find out? Humans utilize facial expressions to reflect their internal state, so it helps when we pay close attention to them.

Making a Good First Impression

Patients are observing us as well, especially at the first meeting. According to a study by professor of behavioral science Alexander Todorov at the University of Chicago, which he covers in his book *Face Value: The Irresistible Influence of First Impressions*, it takes one-tenth of a second for someone to make a first impression, but that's enough time to determine many attributes about one another. People note if you seem kind, pay attention to them, and indicate you can be trusted.

As family caregivers, when we're tired and stressed and in a hurry to get things done, as is often the case, it's easy to drift away from our loved one's needs even though we want to be attentive. Our own preconceptions and assumptions can allow us to miss some important signs from the patient. Keeping our focus on them, when possible, can make a huge difference in our interactions.

Using All of Our Senses

In this chapter I will focus on the various types of nonverbal communication and how to mine them for clues. Often, we don't even think about how important all of our senses are to taking in information—we do it naturally. We use our eyes and ears and nose as well as our sense of touch and even our sixth sense about the emotions in the room to help make interpretations about one another all the time. As we learn to notice and gather more specific information about our family member, we will be better able to decide on the best approach for communicating with them.

For me, observing starts with the overall appearance of a patient from head to toe. I try to do a quick mental scan each time I visit. There are so many areas to observe—it may feel like it's a lot to take in all at once, but you will become more practiced at it over time.

Although as a caregiver it's important to take note of any health or safety issues and address them, for the purpose of this chapter, we will direct our observations to anything that could affect your loved one's ability to communicate or cooperate with you:

» **General health:** Has anything changed since the last time you saw them? Is their skin color normal or pale? Are they moving around as they normally do or are they limping or wincing? Are they steady or shaking? Is their appetite good or are they uninterested?

» **Hygiene:** Do they look presentable or disheveled? Is their clothing appropriate for the time of day? Is their hair reasonably clean and combed? Is there a concerning odor?

» **Seeing and hearing:** Are their eyes bright and are they looking at you with interest? Are they hearing you well or are they struggling?

» **Mood and demeanor:** Do they look alert and interested in talking? Or are they tired, quiet, or tense?

» **Openness to you:** Do they seem to accept your presence in the room or are they irritated or uninterested?

» **Personal space:** Are they comfortable with you standing or sitting close to them or do they appear to be pulling back?

» **Interactions with others:** How do they relate with other family members and other caregivers? Are they generally calm or combative? Do they treat you any differently?

Eye contact is the primary indicator of interest, attention, and involvement. You can rely on that and your loved one's expressions to determine what you can accomplish on any given visit. If they appear to be in pain or discomfort or just in a grumpy mood, it's best to hold off on trying to have long or difficult discussions or starting to implement changes. None of us want to face anything new when we're not feeling our best.

Observing Emotional States

While we note the above, it's also critical to determine how a person is feeling emotionally. It's hard, but helpful, not to jump to conclusions about any of their behavior before we really understand what's going on with them. For example, what appear to be visible signs of anger may have several possible explanations.

Have you ever noticed that some people act out in anger rather than using words? Often that is because they don't know what's going on or what they are feeling—they are simply distraught. In reality, anger often stems from another underlying emotion such as fear or anxiety, or another source such as pain or even just not feeling well.

The same can be true for some people when they are depressed. They may come across as hostile, expressing it as, "Why are you doing that? Why are you putting that there?" But what if they were actually feeling embarrassed rather than angry? Or afraid that their current limitations will go on forever and they may be losing their independence?

It's important to keep in mind that when loved ones come across as mean, they may actually be uncomfortable in some way that they are not communicating. This realization can give us the compassion we need to be more patient with them.

Certain medical conditions—for example, when a person can't breathe well due to asthma or another pulmonary disease—can cause people to develop an angry tone. Again, they may be feeling fear that they can't get enough air, or even that they are going to die. That's such a frightening thought! I tend to say, "Aw, it looks like it's hard for you to breathe right now," so that they know I'm aware of it.

Pain can make one behave outwardly angry or become quick to anger because of the stress it causes. We all are a bit edgy when we are hurting. Pain can also disrupt sleep, which increases irritability.

Fear is a very common emotion that is linked to the fight-or-flight mechanism. Especially when a person has dementia and can't explain with words what is going on or can't understand us, they can act out or become combative. I look for anything that could be causing them discomfort, physically or emotionally. When a person can't use their words, we have to think through all of the possible things that could be bothering them.

Agitation can be a side effect from some medications or be related to sleep deprivation. It can also arise if someone is scared or worried, or even hungry or bored.

Crying can be concerning because it's hard for us to think of our loved ones as being sad. But remember that crying can be a good relief from stress, so we don't necessarily want to interfere with that process. In fact, we want to help them express their emotions so they can release them. Hopefully they will be able to tell you about the feelings that led up to the crying.

Calmness can mean that someone is having a good day. Say, for example, that someone is quietly reading a book. We might assume that it means they are relaxed and happy. But they could instead be trying to distract themselves from worry, or trying to avoid contact with us.

I find it helps to be open to all the clues you notice, then look into all the possible explanations. I will talk in future chapters about how to address some of these issues, but for now, just keep in mind that there may be an underlying reason why your family member is not being receptive, even if they are unwilling or unable to explain to you what it is.

Sometimes, one of these conditions can cause a person to be resistant to every word you say to the point where you feel like leaving the room. While it can help to investigate further, you must proceed carefully. Motivational interviewing, which I introduced in the previous chapter, can be a good technique to use in situations like this. But sometimes a person just needs some alone time, so you might have to return later to be able to get to the bottom of things, even if it's inconvenient.

It's also crucial to observe your own behavior as you interact with your family member, especially in frustrating situations when things aren't going as planned. Don't let yourself get so frustrated that you start to raise your voice. If you start to feel like you can't hold it together any longer, be sure to take a break. Sometimes five minutes away from a stressful situation is enough to re-center yourself and remember that you don't want to increase tension in the relationship; you want to reduce it. You may need to leave and return at a later date with a calmer mindset. As you will read in Chapter 12, it's important for caregivers to take care of themselves, too.

Noticing Out Loud

One technique I have found very helpful is what I call "noticing out loud," which is similar to the "wondering out loud" I mentioned in the previous chapter. When I say, "I'm noticing you do…," I often learn a lot from the responses of my patients. I keep my voice even, without a hint of judgment. This helps them to feel safe, and often they will say, "Yes, I do that because…" which gives me more clarity about their thinking. I find that making statements about what I see is much more effective than directing them or giving immediate solutions. Just observe and notice out loud, which will make your loved one feel that you are interested in their choices.

I try to remember to point out things that are going well, and not just things that concern me. This gets them used to me "noticing" all kinds of things so that they are not put on the defensive. Later I will think about how best to address the problems I see, once they begin to trust that I am there to help, not judge. I will talk more about developing trust in Chapter 6 and nonconfrontational approaches to problem-solving in Chapter 10.

Observing potential safety issues comes up a lot in this chapter because safety is so important! My number one priority with my patients is to help prevent falls and injuries. You are likely caring for a family member who is getting on in years or is simply not as capable as they once were, at least right now. Unsafe environments have the capacity to make a difficult situation so much worse in the blink of an eye.

Using the "Show Me" Technique

Regarding safety, one technique I use is to ask patients to show me how they accomplish everyday tasks. If I want to know about their walking, I ask them to show me the kitchen or the bedroom and observe them on the way. If I want to know about how easily they can move by themselves, I watch how they get up from a chair or bed before we move to another room. If I want to know about their medication management, I ask them to show me their process. Sometimes it could be made a bit easier or safer, so I note that as a topic to address. It's a bit trickier to have the opportunity for them to show me how they take a shower. Usually that means scheduling another visit at their shower time.

It remains important to *hold back any judgment* when you first observe. Oftentimes, a visiting family member only has a short time to see what is going on, so they tend to tell their loved one all of the things that need to be corrected right away. This can be very disheartening for the person, so, if possible, hold off on giving advice in the moment. Maybe during a phone call the next day you could mention one thing that you were unsure of regarding their safety and ask how they felt about it.

Again, the point is not to offer solutions yet, but just to gather information. It may be hard to hold back when you want to fix an issue that has come to light. I have found that in my early interactions with patients if I just *notice without questioning* them, I make better headway in the long run. When they do volunteer an explanation or rationale, I just listen, even though I may disagree with what they are doing and why.

In the next chapter I will talk about how accepting a loved one's worldview, however different from our own, is the best way to keep our interactions patient centered. That does not mean that we don't tell them what we notice; it just means being open to understanding what causes them to do things the way they do. When they feel heard, it makes them more receptive to changes over time.

The following stories demonstrate some ways to begin observing the actions and environment of both your loved ones and yourself:

My Daughters Want Me to Move

I met a woman, Ruth, who lived in a big Victorian home, and noticed that she mainly sat in one room all day with a lot of sun. She used the kitchen, bathroom, and bedroom, but mostly favored one sunny spot. Her daughters thought she would be safer in assisted living and asked for my opinion. After an evaluation I noticed out loud: "It looks to me like you enjoy this nice sunny room."

Ruth responded with, "My daughters want me to move into assisted living but I don't want to go."

I said, "I'll bet if you ever do move, you would want a place with a warm sunny spot like you have now."

I used this observation to show her my awareness of what was important to her, and later I shared the information with her daughters. When she eventually agreed to move, her daughters looked for a new apartment that had a nice sunny spot for her to sit in.

I Wondered How Long It Would Take You

I was so fond of one gentleman, Tom, who lived in a nursing home. He was a sweet soul who seemed content to stay mostly on his own rather than connecting with other residents. One day, as I was about to give him his meds, I knocked on the door to his private room, but there was no answer. Then I noted that his door was locked. I knocked again and there was still no answer. I had to call security for help with the lock. When the door was finally opened, there he was sitting in a chair pulled over near the door. He said, "I wondered how long it would take you to get to me." Tom was just fine and smiled as though he were telling a joke. What did this mean? Was he bored or did he need attention? Even though he stayed in his room most of the time, maybe he was just ready for some more interaction with others. I really wasn't sure. If I'd had time after finishing my round of medication administration, I would have gone back to him and used motivational interviewing to see what was driving this behavior.

It's to be expected that some behaviors will remain a mystery and won't have an obvious meaning or reason behind them, but the key is to remain attentive and observe patterns and preferences so we know when things don't seem quite right.

Note: This event took place in the mid-1980s. Resident rooms in long-term care facilities no longer have locks which avoids a situation like this.

Just a Little Bit

Despite our best efforts, it can be challenging sometimes to observe without judging or jumping to conclusions. I once visited a client named Emma in her home, and when I first went in, I was struck by how dark it was. The shades were shut tightly, the lights were dim, and the whole place felt like a cave to me. I love light—dark places are depressing to me—so I thought maybe I could bring some light into the house to elevate her mood. I asked her if I could open the window shades a bit to make it feel bright and fresh. She said, "Okay, but just a little bit. I can't stand that much light." A few follow-up questions later, I found out that her preference for darkness, which I thought might have been related to depression, was actually a response to her macular degeneration, an eye condition that can occur as people age. Too much bright light was hard on her eyes!

It is so easy to make assumptions, but even when you are intent on observing, it is beneficial to ask questions about what you see so you can try to figure out why things are the way they are.

Remember that when people make decisions, the resulting actions *make sense to them*! You can almost always figure out the "why" behind things, even if you don't understand or agree with the logic yourself.

We'd Like a Professional Opinion

One day a woman called and said, "I went to see my mom over the weekend and I'll be back again next weekend. I don't think she wants anything moved or changed, but it felt like there were a lot of things that were not safe in that house. Can you do an assessment of her situation and let us know how to proceed from here? We'd like a professional opinion."

There were a lot of things I noticed when I went for the home visit, but one chair stood out as being particularly unsafe. The patient, Dorothy, showed me into the kitchen and I asked whether she had eaten breakfast. She put a hand on a chair and was using that for balance while she reached out to grab some items. But the chair was terribly loose and wobbly.

Dorothy didn't seem to notice the unsteadiness at all—it had been that way for so long, I guess, that it didn't strike her as potentially dangerous. As a short-term solution, I asked her if I could swap out the chair for a sturdier one. She quickly agreed, saying, "Oh, sure!" I grabbed another chair from the set that felt more secure. That way she didn't have to change her habits, but she would be using a more stable chair to hold onto. I asked the family to have the wobbly chair repaired to strengthen it so Dorothy could reach for any of them for balance. Just because something works for someone at the moment doesn't mean it's a good solution to the problem in the long term. If she had fallen in the kitchen, she could have badly injured herself.

Now I know you might be thinking—haven't you been telling me to wait to provide solutions to problems after observing them? Normally, yes, it is better to wait. In this instance however, because the issue was one of *safety* and a fall could have *serious consequences*, I intervened right away. If she had resisted, I would have tried bringing her into the process by saying, "Since that chair is wobbly, I wonder what we could do to give you something safe to hold onto." I discuss more tactics for solving problems like this in Chapter 10.

Dangerous conditions are the one thing I will try to solve in the moment if I can because I know how much worse things can get after a fall or other accident. Still, if there is a huge amount of resistance or something requires a more complex solution, I will briefly let a safety issue go but will keep coming back to it over and over until it is solved. I am constantly making mental notes (which I later write down) about issues, but I prioritize safety, especially on the first visit. Fortunately, swapping the chair was an easy fix and she agreed to it right away. By being observant, you can nip some potential issues in the bud and solve problems that could quickly get much worse.

Inch by Inch

One of my patients, Ava, who had dementia, was very accustomed to me being her care manager. We had a good relationship throughout many changes in her life. However, it became necessary for me to introduce her to another provider, Mary, who would become her primary care manager and I would become secondary. I really didn't want to make this change but circumstances demanded it. When I took Mary to introduce her, Ava's lawyer was present as an alternate family member. Ava had complete trust in his judgment. Mary sat at one end of the couch, and I noticed that Ava was sitting at the far other end. The lawyer and I were in chairs across from them. In the midst of all of us talking about the upcoming transition, I noticed Ava doing something I had never seen a patient do before. She moved herself inch by inch closer and closer to Mary! By the time we were done, she was literally sitting beside her. What this meant to me was that she became more and more accepting of Mary as we talked. What a beautiful and loving moment. After we left, I said to Mary, "Did you notice how she moved closer and closer to you? That was her way of saying she accepts you." I never talked with Ava about what I noticed, but that observation meant a lot to all of us, and it was the start of a good relationship between Ava and Mary.

Hopefully you are more aware now of the many nonverbal clues you can take note of that may impact how you care for your loved one. This will help you to get a better sense of their personality and present condition. What I learn from my observations helps me think about what words will be most meaningful when interacting with a patient. How can I help the patient remain calm when discussing their health needs with me?

Imagine yourself in the same condition as your loved one and how you would like someone to approach you. Your instincts will lead you to the answer.

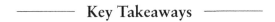

Key Takeaways

» Take the time to become aware of what you are feeling before you enter your family member's environment.
» Set aside your own worries and anxieties before helping them so that you can concentrate fully on observing them.
» Notice nonverbal signs such as facial expressions or behavior.
» Pay attention to all the clues that will help you evaluate their needs, especially their emotional needs.
» Hold off on having difficult discussions if you sense your loved one is not feeling well.
» Gather information by asking them to show you how they accomplish everyday tasks.
» "Notice out loud" things that are going well for them and things that need your attention.
» Focus on creating safe conditions first since falls and accidents can make things so much harder.

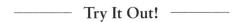

Try It Out!

Try keeping a smile on your face even if you
observe many items that are unsafe and will require
attention. It may make you both feel more relaxed.

CHAPTER FOUR

ACCEPT

As I've talked about in previous chapters, in order to preserve relationships and avoid conflicts, we may have to try a different approach than the one we've been using. If we take on the burden of peaceful communication ourselves, it relieves our loved one and gives us a better chance of producing the outcomes we want.

We often think the way we converse with others is fine and we don't need or want to change our wording. But so do our patients and loved ones! When it comes to conflict, no one wants to think they are the problem, and indeed we may not be in any given situation. We can, however, create peace and cooperation by truly considering another's point of view, which helps them to feel heard.

Have you noticed how much we ourselves want acceptance and yet find it difficult to offer it to others? We often want others to make changes to meet our needs. I think as caregivers this happens more often when we are stressed and have little time to be patient about what has to be done. Acceptance without criticism means so much to all of us. It puts us in a much more cooperative mood, which allows for the development of solutions that work for all.

When people are ill or have diminished capacity, they are more likely to be stubborn or irrational because there are so many things they can no longer control. It doesn't take much for things to get heated. This may be one of the most difficult aspects of family caregiving—remaining calm and keeping the bigger picture in mind when caring for your loved one. It's better to let little things go and save your energy since there may be times when a significant change is important for their health and safety. Identify areas of concern to concentrate your efforts so that you don't become worn out trying to accomplish too much.

At first, you may feel resistant to changing how you speak to your family member. I get it! You're already doing so much, and now you're being asked to think about the very words that come out of your mouth. But keep in mind that once you learn some of these techniques for calm communication, you can use them in your other relationships as well. It's yet another important relationship skill, which builds upon the skills we've already discussed.

Accepting does not mean that we refrain from giving any input with our loved one; it just means we need to let them take more of a lead. Caring for and helping a person does not mean that we are in charge of them. It means that we fill in the parts of their lives that they are unable to handle right now. I remember my own mother telling others how pleased she was to have remained independent even into her late nineties. She seemed unaware of the huge amount that the family was taking care of for her, but that is okay because it means we were able to be a help while allowing her the feeling of autonomy. That feeling was an important need of hers, so we all worked together to promote it.

I used to think that I could help others make a change just by nudging or prompting people, but finally I learned that I needed to alter my approach to have more calm experiences. It changed my life and it can change yours as well.

Avoiding Judgments and Assumptions

Accepting our family member's point of view is a way of showing them respect. It lets them know that we have listened to them and that we care about their preferences. It can help to think about what we would want and how we would react if we were in their shoes. Note that we are not necessarily accepting their behavior, especially if it's inappropriate or unsafe; we are accepting their *point of view* as we work toward positive outcomes for them.

To counter their resistance, we need to remember our goal of peaceful communication. Every discussion that helps a patient or loved one trust us will help them be more open to us. If we lecture or give suggestions too strongly or imply that they are simply wrong, they will begin to reject our "interference," and they will likely stop listening to us. When we're frustrated, it can be easy to blame or overgeneralize, using language like, "Why do you always do that?" This kind of reaction just creates more resistance.

It's also common for caregivers to set unrealistic expectations, focusing on what is still not done or not done right. It's much more helpful to honor our loved one's slow but steady progress.

Even if we're not judgmental in a critical sense, but are just authoritative, it can work against us by pushing others away. Everyone wants to be seen as intelligent and strong and independent, especially those who need to rely on others for help. The best gift we can give to our loved ones is to show them that we truly value their input.

The way to do that is to pay close attention to their feelings and the meaning they ascribe to their daily activities. As I mentioned previously, one of the biggest mistakes we make is assuming other people think the way we think. For example, getting lots of sleep might feel great or horrible, depending on whether it's viewed as restful or lazy. Family visits aren't always happy occasions if the family members don't get along. Recognize that others do not always like the same things you like, and drill down until you truly understand what's going on with them. It's very easy to bring our own assumptions into the picture, or to speculate on what a loved one might be thinking or feeling, but it's much more helpful to be open to the real situation in front of us rather than infusing our own beliefs into it.

Understanding and Honoring Preferences

Each of us is special. We are born with our own unique personalities, and develop as we grow based on training from our parents and the events and circumstances we experience in life. All of us want to be loved and appreciated for who we are.

Partly because they may be from a different generation, family caregivers and the people they are caring for can view things very differently from each other, which can cause friction. Our way always seems best because we have an internal rationale for what we believe or how we behave, but others may have a different rationale that may be just as valid. Our ego somehow wants to get in the way, and we can get caught up in explaining our beliefs to our loved ones at every turn. As we care for them, we need to be careful not to rob them of their uniqueness.

What helps us to be nonjudgmental is to remember that many of our disagreements have to do with preferences. There is rarely a true right or wrong way to do something, just a preference for how it "should be done." Keep in mind that your loved one's life experiences were very different from your own. Even within families, individuals come to see things very differently. Consider some of the following topics that frequently become issues because of the way people view them. These are items with differing interpretations about what "the right thing to do" is.

Since these judgments are usually related to deeply held beliefs about right and wrong, it will be difficult to get someone to change them. Instead, we can change the way we *react* to these tendencies by recognizing that everyone is unique and trying to honor their beliefs. Consider the different interpretations displayed in the following chart.

Topic	Possible Interpretation	Alternate Interpretation
Bedtimes	Early bird	Night owl
Naps	Good for you	Waste of time
Medication	Symptom relief	Unnatural/toxic
Doctor visits	Better to check it out	I'm sure it's nothing
Healthy food	Too expensive	Worth the price
Eating out	A necessity at times	A splurge
Snacking	Bad for you to eat between meals	Keeps blood sugar steady
Fresh air	Good for you	Aggravates allergies
Clean house	Spic-and-span	Good enough
Spending money	Makes life easier	Wasteful
Activities	Good socialization	Too much stimulation
Lights on	Safety	Waste of money

I could go on and on, but the list helps illustrate how differently people think based on their experiences. We need to consider and validate another person's preferences when we can.

Altering How You Communicate

In my family growing up, we were not especially careful with how we spoke to one another and we didn't talk much about feelings, just opinions. This is true of many families. You may not be used to holding back with each other when you have strong opinions or beliefs. Unfortunately, this tendency does not serve family caregivers—or anyone who is in the role of helping others—well.

I personally do not like to be told what to do. Early in my nursing career, this trait helped me to learn a new approach for communicating with patients so that I wasn't in the position of telling them what to do. Ultimately, if someone is capable, they will be more responsive if they are allowed to make their *own* decisions. It's ideal to help a person come up with their own solutions whenever possible. Then we can, if needed, augment their idea to develop a plan that makes everyone comfortable. Of course, this process will likely differ for someone with memory loss, but they too are doing the best they can to cope. In my experience, showing them love, gentleness, and acceptance works well even when they are unable to come up with their own solutions.

I improved my communications skills even more in psychotherapy when I was going through a divorce. Both individual and group therapy gave me tools for dealing with many different personalities. An important paradigm shift for me was realizing that changing *my* communication had a tremendous effect on others. In group, I focused on good coping methods to consider when I was around angry or upset people, including how to speak in a more nonconfrontational manner and how to de-escalate situations when things got tense. I saw how people around me relaxed when I became more aware of their point of view and their motivations. I will talk about some of these techniques in future chapters.

It was not easy for me to change my communication style, and it took me a while, but what an amazing difference! Over the years, I shared what I learned with my children, and as adults they are all quite good at handling situations in a peaceful manner without conflict. You can learn how to do it as well. It might feel impossible at first, but when you see the positive impact it can have on your relationships, you will see that it's worth it.

Let's look at a hypothetical situation and consider how best to handle it.

If a father insists on wearing slippers that everyone agrees are unsafe, a son or daughter might say, "Dad, you have to stop wearing these slippers because you are going to fall!" The approach I would use instead is, "Dad, you just love these slippers, don't you? I wonder if we can find a pair that is similar but safer? How would that be for you?" By phrasing it this way we are saying that we accept what feels good to him and are trying to match that as much as possible while still also considering his safety needs. He may say, "Well, show me some and I'll let you know." That's a start! If he says, "No, these are fine," I would say, "I want your slippers to feel good to you and be safe at the same time. How can we make that happen?" It may take a few go-rounds, but likely he will at least try another pair in the end. It can be done without a conflict.

The starting point is to accept that he likes these familiar and comfortable shoes, and that he doesn't want to get rid of them. That doesn't mean accepting an unsafe situation; it means accepting that he does not initially want to change. When you acknowledge that, it actually opens the door to change. Because you can empathize with him about his preferences, he may allow you to find similar ones with rubber soles that might be safer. When you show someone that you are on their side, that you are really listening to them, and that you accept and acknowledge their feelings and beliefs, they can relax, and relaxation leads to less resistance.

It may take some time, but now that you are aware, you can observe yourself and listen to the wording you typically use with others. Your ideas have to be presented in a way that they can really hear them. Try to be relaxed and calm so that they don't feel the need to react defensively. Notice how much softer the responses are in the right-hand column in this chart.

Instead of This	Try Saying This
Why did you do that?	What made you do that?
You are doing that wrong.	Can I show you another way to do it?
You can't be sleeping all day.	Could you help me with something tomorrow morning around 10:30?
Don't forget your cane!	Your cane seems to really help when you go out, doesn't it?
Oh no, you forgot your pills.	Your pills for yesterday seem to still be in the box.
You have to eat breakfast.	Would just a bite or two work for you?

Instead of This	Try Saying This
Mom, you need to go to the doctor to find out more about your symptoms.	When you go to your doctor, I'm sure you will ask about these symptoms.
Do you *remember* where you put your hearing aid?	I'm looking for your hearing aid.
Don't worry, it's going to all work out.	The future can be scary. Hopefully it will all work out the way you want.
You have to start using a wheelchair.	A wheelchair will be a change. It will help with safety, though.
Dad, you are getting dates mixed up.	There is so much for you to keep track of since you've been sick. Is your calendar big enough for you to write what's coming up?
I'm going to have to start overseeing your banking because you are not paying your bills.	Switching to an online bill pay will give you more time and less worry so you can enjoy yourself more.

Consider the language you are using to make sure others still feel in control. Are you pushing too hard? Are you giving them the information needed to make an intelligent decision on their own? Do you know what is keeping them from making the decision you want them to make? Are you making it easy for them to choose the option that will make you both happy?

I know you will come up with good, creative solutions as well if you can take a breath, stay calm during troubling situations, and consider how your loved one may be feeling. I will talk more about how to do this in the next chapter on empathy.

The following stories offer some ways to offer acceptance and the impact it can have on our interactions:

Are You Sure About That?

My patient Ellen was very frugal and didn't like to waste money on incontinence pads, so she used paper towels. She was having frequent urinary tract infections so I mentioned that disposable pads can be helpful in preventing infections. They absorb the urine rather than letting it linger on your skin. She said, "Really, are you sure about that?" I said it may be worth an experiment to see if pads do help prevent future infections.

Ellen agreed to wear pads for at least a couple of weeks as an experiment. I also mentioned that I would find her ones that were discounted so that she wouldn't have to worry about the money. She wore the pads for many months without an infection. Eventually she did have another UTI and I said, "I wonder why the pads are not helping as much as before?" She told me she had begun using paper towels on top of the pads to save money. She just threw away the paper towel rather than changing the pad. I asked if the cost of an antibiotic and the discomfort of a UTI was worth it. She was reluctant but agreed to start using just the pads again.

I knew that follow-up would be needed every time she considered the cost again but at least all of this was accomplished without an argument. I had to accept that her need to be frugal was very strong.

How many times while reading my description above did you say to yourself, "Paper towels? That's disgusting—what are you doing?!?" I know. Our first instinct is to tell the person they're wrong, or they're being ridiculous, and they should stop immediately. When the same issue comes around again later, families will often say, "We already talked about this, Mom! Using paper towels keeps giving you infections!"

These tactics, though temporarily gratifying, are not the solution to the problem. The solution in this case was to accept that Ellen was frugal to the core and was going to keep trying to think of ways to save money. Often, others' methods are hard for us to understand. It was important for me to help Ellen see how expensive it is to get a UTI. That way, she could still feel like she was saving as much money as possible. By accepting your loved one's point of view, you can use their beliefs to craft messages that will resonate with them. In this scenario, with the right framing, using pads could be thought of as the cheaper solution, and everyone was happy.

Do You Know Who I Am?

One of my patients, Paula, had some dementia. She lived in a beautiful group home. When her sister, Janice, visited her from out of town, I noticed that it was difficult for Janice to witness Paula's decline, especially in what seemed like such a short time. Janice began visiting more often since the family had asked her to oversee Paula's care. When memory loss hits, all family members face the torment of losing the person they once knew so well. The sisters loved each other but could not converse as easily as in the past, which frustrated them both.

Paula's memory loss progressed and she showed signs of depression, which caused her to want to just stay in bed most of the time. As Janice visited Paula more often, it was very difficult for her to see her sister in this condition.

Once, I had just walked in to see Paula when I noticed Janice was visiting. I overheard their conversation. Janice said to her sister, "Hi, do you know who I am?" Paula said, "No," which was so hurtful to Janice.

After that visit, I went back into Paula's room to talk with her and noticed two things. Paula barely opened her eyes all the way, so it was unclear if she was able to pay attention. I called her name and asked her to let me see her eyes. She opened them and looked at me. I smiled and said, "Hi, I'm your friend Joan. Once you and I had a great trip together to Annapolis to enjoy all the sailboats. I know you used to love sailing your boat." She perked up and said, "I know, I know." We had a short discussion afterwards. She may not have actually remembered me, but she was aware that I was someone who cared about her and talked about something she enjoyed in life. Sometimes that's the most that can be expected.

I later explained to Janice how I was able to witness a positive reaction from her sister and said I hoped her next visit would be that way as well. I encouraged Janice to try something similar to what had worked for me. I let her know that I understood how tempting it was to want to know if Paula could still recognize her, but that asking might cause disappointment for both of them. I advised her that "even if Paula doesn't remember your name or face, she can sense that you're someone who loves her. Just keep showing your love for her and she will be pleased with your visits."

Accepting changes in our loved ones can be sad, but with different communication tools, a sense of joy can occur as well. Life is changing all the time, yet many of us try very hard to keep it the same. When our loved one changes due to illness, their personality may change dramatically and we will miss the healthy person they once were. Despite this, rather than remain in denial—a tempting and common reaction—it's so meaningful to accept who they are today. I think most of us would want to be accepted even if we lost an arm or broke a hip or became disfigured in some way. Even though we want to be accepting, our own sadness may interfere. This is again the time to look for the person within who has value and importance and who needs you. Accepting is a way to show your love for them.

Once you accept a situation, it benefits you as well. Fighting against something that is not going to change does not help us. In fact, it only frustrates us. It is difficult to let go of the way things used to be, but until you accept the way things are now, you can't help make the current situation as good as it can be. By asking questions that she didn't really want to hear the answer to ("Do you remember me?"), Janice was setting up the relationship for failure and disappointment. If she could let go of the past, she could see that the best way to serve her sister and herself was to walk in with a smile and shower her sister with warmth and love despite her deteriorating memory.

Very often, accepting involves disappointment for us. It's important to recognize that we need to grieve the loss before we can move on from it. Losing pieces of a loved one—their memory, their speech, their ability to walk—comes with its own kinds of grief. It doesn't help that some of these pieces of grief are coming in advance of a possible further grief: their passing. If our loved one is fortunate, they may heal and we can enjoy their personality again. If they are unable to heal, we need to be there for them even if it makes us sad.

Bugs in My Ears

My patient Sarah was living independently but over-medicating herself with anti-anxiety meds. My service was initiated to manage her medications. I asked if she would allow a pill organizer box so we would know exactly what she takes each week. It would also let us know when to order refills. Surprisingly, she agreed. After a week of consistent med doses, she began feeling like she had bugs in her ears. She became more and more agitated, and her aides and their supervising nurse thought she was going crazy and should be taken to the emergency room.

I knew from experience that simply telling her "There are no bugs in your ears" was likely to increase her agitation even more. She was feeling them, and that feeling was important to recognize, whether imagined or real. I listened to Sarah and said, "I would hate that feeling."

If I hadn't accepted what she was saying was true for her (even though everyone else thought it was nonsense), I wouldn't have been able to figure out the real problem. Even if your family member is expressing something in a strange way, it doesn't mean there isn't a real, underlying issue. Accept that this is what it feels like to them, even if it doesn't make sense to you. Resisting and pushing back will be frustrating for you both and will not elicit the response that you want.

I did some research and found that one of Sarah's meds could cause a sensation of "having bugs in the ears" if it is decreased too rapidly. Though she was given the correct dose that week, it was apparently much lower than what she had been taking on her own. The solution, per her physician, was to increase the dose again until she calmed down and then lower it again more gradually. No ER visit was required.

I was reminded again to always pay attention to what someone is telling me unless I find out otherwise. I had never heard of a drug causing that type of feeling in one's ears but was very relieved when I learned about it so we could find a solution. Sarah was also relieved because someone listened, and the "bugs in ears" feeling eventually went away.

Someone Stole My Scarf!

On another visit, my patient Terry, who had memory loss, yelled, "Someone stole my scarf! I've looked everywhere, and I can't find it!" She was quite angry and agitated. I replied, "Oh, I hate when that happens." I showed acknowledgement by saying, "I'll help you find it." Instead, most people are likely to say, "Mom, no one is stealing from you!" It's a natural response, but this may frustrate her and make her feel more alone and invalidated. I asked her what color the scarf was so that I could keep an eye out for it. Again, recognize and accept what this feels like to her. Likely it will show up before long and no argument need occur.

"Someone is stealing from me" and "Someone took my things" are very common statements from someone who has memory loss. When an item isn't where they think it should be—maybe because they moved it and forgot or perhaps it's actually been gone for years—it feels natural to them to assume someone took it. Their brains are trying to interpret the situation when they can't figure out what's happening. When a family member blocks this line of reasoning with "No one is stealing from you mom!" or "You're not missing anything," they become agitated. If something disappeared from your house, what would you think happened to it? That it just disappeared? No! Of course someone took it!

Instead, I honor their feelings. They certainly *feel* like something is missing, and that feeling is valid. I usually say something like, "I can keep an eye out for it." I'm not telling them they are right or wrong; I am letting them know that I am hearing what they are saying, and what they are saying matters to me. I want them to know that I'm on their side and I will be a help to them. The more you shut someone down, the less they'll tell you.

———————

Accepting others without judgment can lead to much more peaceful interactions with them. Learning to accept anything new or different is a process. It may not happen overnight, but we can work toward it. Consider that as hard as it is for us to accept things we don't like, our patients or loved ones with diminished capacities are also having to accept many changes that are hard for them. We have this in common with them, and this realization can give us empathy for what they are facing. The things they have to accept often involve difficult and frustrating losses such as losing the autonomy that comes with driving or not having the energy to attend important events such as weddings. None of us like to think of these things happening to us, but eventually they will, if we're fortunate enough to live a long life. We will want our caregivers to be understanding about our desire to remain in control or at least have the opportunity to give input about our needs and desires for as long as possible.

——— Key Takeaways ———

- » Keep in mind your goal of peaceful communication.
- » Accept your loved one's worldview without judgment.
- » Don't assume that others see things the way you do.
- » Identify areas of concern to concentrate your efforts.
- » Remember that many of our differences have to do with preferences, not right or wrong thinking.
- » Try to stay relaxed and calm so your family member doesn't feel the need to react defensively.
- » Accept their memory loss without testing them. "Do you remember?" can feel like a test.
- » Always recognize that their sensations are real to them.
- » Help them look for a lost article rather than denying that it is lost. Remember that it is lost to them.

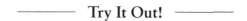

Try It Out!

Learn to accept what your loved one is saying even when it doesn't make sense to you. See how much calmer they become when you trust that their feelings are real.

CHAPTER FIVE

SHOW EMPATHY

In the last few chapters, I've offered some ways we can learn more about our loved ones, which can help make caregiving go more smoothly. In particular, I've focused on the importance of listening, observing, and accepting their worldview. Starting with this chapter, we will shift our focus to ourselves, and take a look at how our reactions and responses can soothe our family members and help them to feel heard.

The tool we will rely on most heavily is our empathy for them and their current situation, whether it's a short-term injury or a chronic illness. When we summon up our feelings of compassion, and respond from that place in our hearts, it will make our family members feel that we are there for them. When they feel supported, they will be much more likely to be cooperative.

Whether or not you have chosen the role, you have been called to be of service to your loved one. There is no better tool available to you as a caregiver than your own feelings for your family member who may be in distress. My favorite definition of empathy comes from Dr. Brené Brown, a research professor at the University of Houston who studies courage, vulnerability, shame, and empathy. She says, "Empathy is simply listening, holding space, withholding judgment, emotionally connecting, and communicating that incredibly healing message of you are not alone."

Many people confuse the terms sympathy and empathy, which are closely related. Sympathy involves looking at a situation from our perspective, such as the times when we feel pity for someone else's misfortune—perhaps a homeless person on the street. It is a more limited emotion. When we feel sympathy, we are usually looking at someone from afar but have less personal involvement.

By contrast, empathy involves connecting emotionally, which starts with trying to *understand* the other person's feelings and why they may be having them. As I mentioned in Chapter 3, to figure out what's going on with our loved one on any given day, we can read their nonverbal cues: facial expressions, tone of voice, and behavior. In this chapter I will talk about how to use your imagination to determine what your family member might be going through as they recover from an injury, learn to cope with a disability, or suffer through an illness, and how you can help them feel more supported by choosing your words carefully.

Empathy is critical to the work that we do as caregivers, as it can lead us to act more compassionately, even when we're frustrated or tired. When we *feel* more loving toward someone, we tend to *act* in a way that is more loving. This can go a long way toward reducing conflict and make the caregiving experience much more rewarding. As Brené Brown further explains, "Empathy is feeling *with* people, which fuels connection."

Probably because I am emotionally sensitive, I have always been naturally empathetic, but I recognize that it's more of a struggle for some people. As you are learning the communication tips offered here, especially if they are new to you or you have a complex relationship with the person you are caring for, you may find it awkward, uncomfortable, and frustrating at first. It is important for you to know that these techniques will come more naturally to you over time. Your intention to be more loving will motivate you to get past your initial frustrations with your loved one to see what they might be feeling.

My understanding of others, especially when they are suffering, deepened as a result of my early training. My instructors stressed that we would learn empathy best by being placed in situations that patients experience to know what it might feel like.

One teaching method my school used involved role-playing sessions. We were asked to stand next to a hospital bed with an imagined patient lying in the bed who might have bandages on or IVs attached. We were told the medical issues involved and were asked to demonstrate how we would respond to the situation. That made us think through our side of the conversation, and then the instructor would help us choose better words.

In our classes we took turns being pushed in a wheelchair or placed on a stretcher and even had someone shave our legs as would sometimes be necessary for a patient before surgery. The training was very effective—it gave us a much better understanding of what it feels like to be a patient than just talking about it did. At the same time, it gave us a taste of the caregiving experience as well when we were the ones transferring the patient, pushing the wheelchair, and so on.

I've always felt so fortunate to be a nurse because I learned these techniques early in my life. Being able to tune in to what's going on with others has enhanced all my relationships throughout my life, not just the ones with my patients.

My communication skills continued to advance throughout my career, mainly through trial and error as I worked to make my patients feel cared for. In the hospitals and facilities where I worked, I also had many fine supervisors and mentors who taught me how to interact with patients who were not feeling their best.

Using Your Imagination

Have you ever had a time where you found it hard to relate to someone else's situation until you went through something similar yourself? If you've noticed that it's easier for you to have empathy for your children than for your aging parents, it may be because you were a child at one point in your life and so you can relate. But since you have not yet been a senior, it's more difficult to imagine.

There is nothing like having a difficult or painful experience yourself to give you an understanding of the struggle involved and the emotions it brings up, especially fear and anxiety. Often when this happens, we are humbled, and we resolve to do better.

Throughout my career I have encountered doctors who were hospitalized for various medical conditions, and they all told me they gained "new insight" from their experience and realized they needed to be more empathetic to patients. It's impossible to completely put ourselves in other people's shoes to get that personal experience, and we can't undergo everything that others are going through. But we can at least try to imagine what it must be like for them by intuiting what it would be like for us if we were in the same situation.

Becoming Curious

I mentioned previously that we can use the technique of motivational interviewing to learn what motivates patients to become more understanding of their needs. Being curious is the best stance to have if we truly want to understand people and develop more loving feelings for them. Compassion—caring enough to take action to be helpful to others—is a natural extension of empathy. When we ask the right questions in the right way, out of genuine concern and curiosity, we can gain valuable information that can help us support our loved ones.

I like to keep in mind that at any time I may be the one who requires assistance, and I know I would want my caregiver to inquire about what I'm thinking or what my concerns are. Empathy, compassion, and curiosity are three of our most powerful and important emotions and can serve as strong antidotes to the suffering of others.

Tapping into Your Empathy

When people don't feel well, they tend to complain a lot, which can wear on us over time and cause us to lose our patience. Our responses have the power to calm our patients or loved ones or to stir them up. I have learned that the careful use of words that show our compassion toward them can elicit a much more satisfactory outcome. Once I discovered this truth, I saw it as a blessing because I had a tool I could rely on that made every interaction more positive.

Some people, especially those with social anxiety, feel concern for others but don't know how to express it. They aren't sure what to say or how to respond in a way that demonstrates their caring feelings. There are many ways to learn the empathy required for more peaceful communication such as through reading, taking classes, listening to podcasts, or choosing to be around nonjudgmental people and listening to the ways they speak to others. One book in particular I recommend is titled *Born for Love: Why Empathy is Essential—and Endangered* by Maia Szalavitz.

It does take time and effort to increase your capacity for empathy, as learning any new skill does, but it can save you time in the long run by reducing friction.

The frustration involved in conflict drains your energy. By contrast, witnessing your loved one's cooperation when they are relaxed and happy is uplifting. It improves your energy as well as theirs. When they can see that you care, and are at least trying to understand, it will be easier for them to appreciate your efforts on their behalf. If you are thoughtful in your responses so that the tension does not escalate, you will be able to get on the same page more easily. Working as a team to solve problems will make your relationship so much more enjoyable.

The table that follows shows some sample wording that may help you arrive at better outcomes when interacting with your family member. As you read each example, notice how you feel when you read the more typical responses that, while they may be accurate, dismiss the person's feelings. Do they make you tense up? That's how our loved ones feel when we are short with them and use statements that shut down their communication rather than encourage them to open up more so we can better understand their needs or concerns. Now notice how you feel when you read the empathetic responses that acknowledge and address their feelings. Do they make you feel calmer and more relaxed?

Patient	Typical Response	Empathetic Response
No one cares about what I think.	Of course we care about what you think!	What would help you feel that we cared about your thoughts?
I don't want to be in a wheelchair.	You have to be in a wheelchair because you are so weak now.	What would it be like for you to be in a wheelchair just for now?
I am not moving and that is that.	You have to move— you're not safe here!	You feel strongly about staying in your home, don't you?
The food here tastes terrible.	Really? It looks so good to me.	What would make the food taste good to you?
I feel so cold.	The heat is up, and you have lots of blankets on you.	Would another blanket help?
I am so tired.	Dad, you can't still be tired, you've been sleeping all day!	I wonder what is making you feel so tired?
You never told me about that before.	But Mom, I called you yesterday and told you.	Oh, wow, it's a good thing we are talking about it now then.
That doctor doesn't know what she is talking about.	Now Mom, she was just trying to let you know what's going on.	What were you hoping to hear from her?
I've lost all my dreams of the future since this illness.	Well, things change and we have to live with it.	Tell me about your dreams.

Dealing with Emotional Numbness

Even if you are naturally very caring, you may have times where you're unable to summon up much feeling for your loved one. This may be the result of cumulative days, weeks, months, or even years of managing caregiving responsibilities that are often unrecognized, seemingly endless, emotionally demanding, and physically exhausting. Sleep loss, in particular, is strongly associated with lack of empathy and can result in miscommunications that can lead to conflict.

I have felt compassion fatigue myself, and it was embarrassing to think I had lost my typical level of patience. I didn't want others to know how I felt. I just kept going until it became too much. Many of you may be in that situation right now. What can you do?

In Chapter 12, I will talk much more about the need for caregivers to practice self-care so they don't get to the point of burnout. Taking a break when you feel your empathy decreasing is imperative. Pushing through these feelings instead of asking for help can lead to substandard care, fighting or snippiness, and other bad outcomes. Even if you can only take short breaks occasionally, that is better than nothing. Breaks can help change your perspective. Step back from the situation, take a deep breath, rest, and find a way to ease your tension. Your caring feelings will return if you put yourself first and take care of some of your own needs for a change.

Here are some stories that demonstrate the ways you can show empathy with your family member:

It's Not Hot Enough

One of my patients, Harry, had some issues with the temperature of the water when he was being showered. It can be very difficult for patients to accept that someone else is in control, so as caregivers we need to help them feel more in charge. One day when I was helping his wife, Elise, shower him, Harry said, "The water is not hot enough." She replied, in what is often the response, "It is plenty hot." This angered him. Unfortunately, she was denying his feelings instead of listening to him.

I told her, "He doesn't feel that it is hot enough, though," so that she would think about and understand his point of view a bit more. My guess was that Elise was worried about burning him and that her statement was likely coming from a place of caring, not dismissal. I checked the temperature of the water myself and told her it was safe to make it a bit warmer.

Once she did so, he responded happily, "Now that's better!" Of course, we must be careful not to burn people, but we also have to listen to them and rely on their judgment (unless there is a cognitive impairment that could affect their judgment). If I felt it was not safe to increase the temperature, I still would not have dismissed his feelings. I would have tried to find another way to make him feel warmer—perhaps I would have asked him whether using a warm towel on his lap (he was sitting on a shower chair) might help.

It is so important to tune in to how things feel for your loved one, even when we do not necessarily agree. Next time you are in the shower, try making a small adjustment away from your normal temperature—it can make quite a difference over the course of a few minutes. Now imagine if you could no longer shower on your own and someone else was not listening to your preferences. This is where our empathy comes into play. Trying to understand from their point of view can help us offer good solutions without the struggle. As I discuss in detail in Chapter 9, it also helps to be flexible in these situations, as long as everyone remains safe.

She's Very Confused Today

A man named Hank contacted me and asked for my advice and assistance with a situation. His mother, Gena, had been falling frequently and seemed to be getting much weaker since she'd had a UTI two weeks prior. Hank's sister had spoken with their father, George, several times that day to try to get him to take her to the ER for an evaluation. George declined to take her since he already had a doctor's appointment scheduled for her on the following day.

I called George and asked how his wife was feeling. He told me, "Gena has been ailing the past few days. She's just getting weaker and weaker." Trying to be positive, he also mentioned that she seemed to be a bit better during the day but seemed sicker in the evening. However, he then admitted, "She is very confused today, though, and sometimes looks as though she could faint."

Hank had also told me that his parents were expecting holiday visitors, and he had arranged for a carpet cleaning company to be there that day. George said they had to be out of the house for a few hours, so he and the caregiver planned to take Gena to Starbucks and just wait there until the cleaning was over. It was a very stressful time for him between caring for his increasingly sick wife and dealing with the preparation of the house for visitors.

I timed my next call for when I knew they would be at Starbucks and suggested that George might as well take her to the emergency room for an evaluation since they had some time to kill. I also mentioned that if she got worse and he wound up having to call 911 for support, it would be quite upsetting for her.

I told him that if Gena stabilized at the ER, they could send her home right away, but at least they could have blood work done and maybe an IV for hydration. He was still very much inclined to wait until the next day to deal with her condition. Undaunted, I continued my gentle pressure campaign by explaining that if she got any weaker, he might not be able to care for her himself. (The caregiver was not there at night, so no one would be available to help him.) He replied that he would keep a close eye on her. I told him I thought it was likely that he might have to call 911 in the middle of the night and suggested that he should sleep in his clothes just in case. That really concerned him, so he finally agreed to drive her to the ER. She was admitted with severe dehydration and a worsening UTI, which had returned. Her kidneys were also at risk, so it was good that I persisted.

Imagining what it was like for this husband under so much stress helped me to consider the issue from his point of view. George had a lot on his plate already, and I was asking for something that he felt might not have been necessary. Oftentimes we become upset with someone who seems to be uncooperative, but understanding their motivations can make such a difference. He was only trying to simplify his life by waiting until the next day and did not think in the moment that going to the ER was totally necessary. That might have been true, except that Gena sounded ill enough to me to warrant the trip. He was relieved when she was admitted to the hospital since they could care for her and give her fluids and a different antibiotic by IV. She started improving the next day and was able to be released before long to enjoy her visitors.

Not Old Enough to Need Care Yet

Charles had been hospitalized with pneumonia and a possible stroke. Being sick was incredibly frustrating for him since he lost the independence he was used to. Once he was fairly recovered, he agreed to be sent to a rehab center for strengthening, which was very helpful to him. Though he worked hard in therapy, he reached a point of no further progress and was ready to be discharged. He was quite happy to finally be going back to his senior apartment.

Unfortunately, he now required a wheelchair and lacked the strength to transfer himself from his wheelchair to his bed. Since the apartment he lived in prior to rehab did not have any aides or other staff to help him with these transfers, his family insisted that he move into an assisted living apartment instead so that he would have adequate help. He became obstinate and stopped discussing the issue with them. He had not even considered the possibility that he would not be going back to his own comfortable home after rehab and was upset that it was being proposed.

The family called me to help convince Charles to go into an assisted living facility. He was financially secure enough to afford it but was very frugal and wanted to save his money in case he needed it later. He was 88 years old, so to everyone else it appeared like a good time to use these funds, but he did not see it that way. He did not feel, as he described it, "old enough to need care yet."

I sat down with him to discuss things while trying to keep an open mind so I could understand his point of view. After talking with him, I realized just how much his senior independent apartment meant to him. He was relaxed there, had friends nearby, and it was less expensive than assisted living. I also discovered that the reason his family had insisted on moving him to another facility was that he had refused to have any kind of care in his apartment. A situation where Charles had no care at all was unrealistic and unsafe, but he stood very firm about his wishes. I understood where he was coming from—it can be remarkably difficult for anyone to accept that they are no longer capable of living day to day without assistance.

I told him I would support him returning to his apartment instead of the assisted living, but that option would require him to accept help there. He said, in no uncertain terms, "No." I reminded him that it was his decision to make as he was of sound mind, then asked if he would talk with me about how he imagined his life once he was discharged. He said, "I just want to go home." Again, I explained that I wanted to help him accomplish that, but a safe discharge plan was essential, and I just wanted him to walk me through how his discharge would be safe and he would make himself comfortable and able to live in his old place.

As he thought things through, he started talking about paying someone to get his groceries, which was a good start. He also said he was willing to pay someone for regular cleaning of the apartment. I offered him encouragement by telling him that he was thinking in a positive direction, and that his ideas so far would definitely contribute to his comfort and safety.

I asked him if he was currently transferring from his wheelchair into his bed independently at the rehab facility. He said, "No, but I'm getting stronger." I replied, "What would it be like if you continued with help from an aide at home just until you got strong enough to return to the independence you once had?" I suggested that, "Continuing that strength training at home until you are stronger could be a great option temporarily to keep you from returning to the hospital." I knew that returning to the hospital was a big concern for him, so I used my understanding of his motivations to nudge him to make a plan that would avoid an outcome he did not want.

I told him, "You have transitioned beautifully from the hospital to rehab, and now the next step in your recovery could be home if you agree to have help." I explained to him that in the past, people used to be kept in the hospital much longer until they were stronger before they were released back home, but health care had changed. Now, most people utilize a rehab center, then discharge either to home with a home health care aide or to an assisted living facility. I asked him what he felt was the healthiest option for right now. He answered, "Home, of course."

Again, I offered him the only safe plan for returning home: "Okay, so an aide and a physical therapist at home would be acceptable to you to continue your strength training?" He said, "I guess I have to." I told him, "I bet you have made many tough decisions in your life even when you didn't want to. This seems like the best option for now." Since he was willing to accept the aide and physical therapist and his plan was safe, I became an advocate for his choice. I let him know, "Your family still insists on assisted living for you, but I am willing to help them understand how important going back home is to you. You can share with them all the decisions you have made to keep yourself safe and comfortable, and I will fully support you in your choices."

The family was not thrilled but were glad to hear he would accept help at home. Their fear was that he would cancel the help once he was home. I agreed that he might want to but told them that I trusted that he would realize that by working hard in physical therapy he might be able to safely cancel the help as soon as he got strong enough, which would motivate him to make that happen.

The use of empathetic prompting (asking questions with the intent to understand) shifted both his and the family's perspectives. He agreed to safety measures he had resisted in prior discussions so he could remain at home as he desired because he understood that his family was just trying to keep him safe and comfortable. The family was at least temporarily satisfied with the outcome once they realized how much his home really meant to him. I am mindful that situations can change rapidly, especially with aging adults, and all solutions have to be revisited depending on how things play out, but since there were no longer any immediate concerns about safety, we could at least proceed forward until the situation changed. If Charles fired the help, for example, we would have had to rethink the situation.

———————

It is often said that one of the best ways to be happy in life is to be of service to others. Professional caregivers are trained to imagine themselves in someone else's place, especially someone who is not feeling well, so they can empathize with them. As a family caregiver, identifying with and seeking to understand your loved one's trials and tribulations will go a long way toward maintaining peace with them. As you become more curious about their point of view and begin to understand better what they are feeling, your empathy will increase. In addition, your interest and concern will demonstrate to them that you genuinely care about their happiness and well-being. You may be amazed at the outcome when you start to use some of the techniques in this chapter and see things begin to change from frustration to cooperation.

As spiritual author Mary Davis says, "We can't heal the world today, but we can begin with a voice of compassion, a heart of love, an act of kindness." Treasure your innate ability to feel deeply for others and nurture it. It is a beautiful gift and using it will help to calm and smooth situations of all kinds, not just with those you are caring for.

──────── **Key Takeaways** ────────

» Imagine how a given situation might feel to your family member.

» Be curious and ask questions to learn more about what they need emotionally.

» When someone is highly resistant to change, sometimes a first step is to allow them their choice, but only if they agree to safety measures.

» Ask a loved one to walk you through how they would handle specific scenarios to reduce resistance to having an aide or implementing safety measures.

» Try to understand your loved one's point of view, as it will help you be more empathetic.

» Communication skills can be learned through reading, classes, groups, etc.

» Use kind words that show you care about what your loved one is going through.

» Use empathetic responses to encourage them to open up rather than shut down.

» Take physical and mental breaks when possible to maintain your empathy.

──────── **Try It Out!** ────────

Try withholding judgment and see if you note a more receptive reaction from the person you are caring for.

CHAPTER SIX

BUILD TRUST

When we show respect, take the time to listen, validate concerns, and show empathy to our loved ones, we can build up their trust in us over time. We can then leverage the strength of our relationship with them to encourage them to make changes. This is true even for changes that are contrary to their own wishes, but essential to their health or well-being. By being honest and true to our word, we are often able to overcome their initial resistance and find a solution that works for everyone.

Trusting someone means that you believe them. You sense that they are reliable and speak the truth—you have no reason to doubt them. When you trust someone, it allows you to let go of some of the need to control things. If they tell you they will handle something, you know they will. Trust relies on consistency in both words and actions.

Importantly, the opposite is true as well—when there is no trust, people will feel the need to control and they will worry. They may feel that the solutions presented to them by others are not in their best interest, chalking it up to selfish motivations ("My daughter only wants to move me so it's easier for her."), misrepresentation ("These aides say they care about me but I don't think they actually do."), or lack of ability ("That doctor doesn't know what he is talking about.").

Building the Relationship

When visiting patients, I very much go out of my way to try to make a connection with them—to see them as people, not just patients. It's important to me to find out what they love, and what is meaningful to them. Once I find out, I engage them about it even if I don't have a particular interest in it. I enjoy hearing about what people used to do for work or for hobbies when they were younger. Enthusiasm is infectious, and it makes my job more interesting to understand why their passion is important to them.

When you are caring for a family member, you can create opportunities to get to know them better. Ask them to share more about their life and interests or even what they used to do for work or for fun. You may be surprised how much you don't know about them, and how much you can still learn from them. If you take the time to have these conversations, it will enhance the trust between you because they will see that you truly care about them. If they see you as someone who enjoys them and respects them, it will go a long way toward building trust. It also makes it easier for them to follow your nudges in the future to help them solve problems.

Building Emotional Trust

In addition to building trust on a practical level, it's important to build emotional trust with our patients. So how do we show our loved ones we're on their side? As I've said, I find that when I stay calm, show interest, and look into my patients' eyes, they begin to relax. Then I work on strengthening our connection by smiling at them to convey warmth and encouragement. I take my time with them, which lets them know that what they have to say is important to me. I ask questions, and then try hard to stay nonjudgmental about whatever they share so that they see I have their best interest at heart.

I also allow myself to be a little vulnerable with them when it feels appropriate. I let them know that I sometimes struggle with the same thing they are struggling with. This acknowledgement that we're all human helps them to be more open with me, which further cements our relationship. The more I understand what they need, the better I can care for them.

It may seem counterintuitive, but if you want others to trust you, you need to trust them first. This means giving someone the benefit of the doubt and believing that what they say is real to them. Remember the story in Chapter 4 called "Bugs in my Ears"? By putting my trust in Sarah and believing her when no one else did, I showed her that I was reliable. From that point forward, she trusted me in everything else we did. For my part, I continued to believe her side of things unless I found out otherwise.

Trust is not a one-way street—building trust in a relationship means building trust in each other, not just asking your patient or loved one to put their trust in you.

Recognizing That Distrust Comes with the Territory

If you are caring for a family member, they already know you, but they may need time to trust you in your new role. As I've mentioned, after being "in charge" for so long, it can be very difficult for aging adults to turn over the control of their lives to someone younger, even when it's clear they need help. Generational issues can arise and complicate matters.

If you and your relative were close before their illness or injury, you may be surprised when they start to balk at your suggestions. This can be quite upsetting since you know your motives are pure. It may come as a surprise to you to learn that many older people are naturally distrustful, even if that was not a typical personality trait for them in the past. Some of these new barriers to trust between family members are predictable in caregiving situations:

- » They may feel that you're too busy or rushed to listen to them, so they don't have confidence that you'll know what they really want.
- » They may be concerned that family members are talking about them behind their back.

» They may be distrustful of all caregivers—family members or outsiders—because they don't want to be told what to do.

» They may be tired of surgeries, treatments, and medicines, or feel that they are unnecessary, so they may distrust those who are involved in making decisions about further interventions.

» They may be conservative with money and worry that caregivers will try to get them to spend it on items they don't really need.

Understanding what you're up against, and why, can help. Seniors feel more vulnerable than usual when they require your assistance, especially if it's new to them. Listening, observing, accepting, and being empathetic helps them know that you care about them and their needs. They will begin to feel more secure over time as you demonstrate reliability and predictability. It will help them to see that you are on their side.

Tips for Earning a Person's Trust

There are many different things you can do to earn a person's trust. I have touched on several in previous chapters. Here are some additional tips to keep in mind:

» Be open and honest, and commit to working on the relationship, realizing that it is central to the care you are providing.

» Talk to one another and listen attentively. Resist the urge to jump in with suggestions right away.

» Create new positive experiences together as often as you can.

» Keep and follow through on any commitments you make.

» Admit your mistakes and apologize.

» Give the person you are caring for the benefit of the doubt whenever possible.

If you make family members feel comfortable and safe in these ways, they will be more inclined to share with you what they are thinking and feeling. This will create an opportunity for cooperative problem-solving.

The following stories show how it's possible to build a trusting relationship with your loved one:

Today's Not a Good Day

This story is about how small gains can lead to bigger ones over time. You don't have to intervene too quickly or try to make big changes right away.

I went to my new client's apartment building for a first-time appointment. Her name was Ann, and I was told in advance that she was very resistant to anything new. I used my cell phone to call her from the lobby. She answered but said, "I don't feel well. Today's not a good day, so you can't come."

I said, "Oh that's fine, we don't have to meet today. May I come up for a second and can you crack the door a bit just so we can see what one another looks like?"

Ann hesitated, but then said it was okay. I went up to her door and knocked. She came to the door and we talked for a moment. When I was about to leave, she said, "It's okay, you can come in."

I responded, "Thank you, but I told you we would just meet briefly like this so I will come back later." Then, as we had agreed, I left for the day. I didn't want to get into a question of trustworthiness or to have her suspect that this was just a trick for me to get in that day.

None of the tools or methods in this book are about tricking people. Instead, they are about being honest and trustworthy and building a relationship. By starting with trust, you can build a foundation that will keep growing over time. When she invited me that day after she had already said it was not a good day, if I had gone in, she might have always secretly suspected that I had manipulated her, and this could have led to issues down the road.

Also, importantly, who am I to judge whether she was trying to avoid me or just not feeling well that day? It is always best to assume the most positive motivation for a person's actions. I am well aware that a patient may push me away because they are afraid to meet with someone new, but they may also legitimately not feel well. Trust and respect go both ways. I try to keep in mind what the situation is like for the patient to help me adjust to their needs.

You're Here Again

Carolyn was a woman in her forties who was suffering with emotional issues. She was slated for release from the psychiatric unit of the hospital, but every time her actual discharge day came around, she became agitated and uncooperative. She would have something similar to a panic attack and begin acting out, yelling, and actively resisting the staff. The hospital staff was able to calm her down using medication and would continue to care for her for a while longer. Since this happened on every attempted discharge day, her family asked the hospital if they could pay privately for her to stay longer in the hospital, and the staff agreed. This scenario occurred two more times, and finally the hospital stated that she must be discharged to a different facility.

The family called me to see if I could possibly help their daughter be discharged peacefully. I agreed but said that I needed some time to establish a trusting relationship with her. I talked with the psychiatrist and hospital staff, and it was decided that I would be invited to her individual care plan team meeting every week with multiple doctors and staff members.

I arrived at the next team meeting and the patient asked immediately who I was and what I was doing there. I told her, "I'm a nurse, and I am learning about the process here at the hospital." Both statements were true. I may not have expressed the full intent of why I was there, but I was completely honest.

The second week, I attended again. The patient said, "Joan Foust, you're here again!" I was a little surprised that she remembered my full name, but I later found out that she had an extraordinary memory. I said, "Yes, I'm going to come for a little while. I'm still learning this process." Still all true. At the end of that meeting, I said to her, "I'm going downstairs to get a snack. Do you want anything?"

She said, "I want to come with you, but they won't let me."

Since she tended to act out when she left the unit, they had restricted her movement. I told her, "If you really want to go with me downstairs, I think we can do that if you agree to stay calm while we're there."

She agreed, and when I asked permission, her nurse agreed as well, so I signed her out, and took her downstairs. We both had a snack and a drink, which gave her a reprieve from what she had come to think of as her "jail." Fortunately, the journey was without incident. I had trusted her in this scenario, and she had proven herself. She was beginning to understand that I could potentially make things better for her, but only if everything remained calm. Our trust for each other was building slowly but surely.

We came back up and went to her room. I noted that she had no telephone. When I asked her about it, she said they wouldn't let her have one. I said, "Oh, I'd hate that. I love having a phone. Someday you'll be in a place where you will have your own phone. I can help you find a place when you're ready." This was my way of sowing a seed, giving her something to imagine and look forward to, even if it was small. She had already seen that I could get her out of her "jail," and now I was telling her about another potential benefit of relying on me for help.

The third time I went to the meeting, I discovered that she played the piano and that there was one on the unit. After the meeting, I asked her to play the piano for a bit, and she did. She had been a classical pianist, but the medication she was on made her fingers stiff so she said she didn't play as well as she had in the past. Still, she seemed to enjoy it, and we created yet another shared positive experience together.

I continued to paint a picture for her of a better world outside of the hospital: "Imagine what it would be like to find a home that has a piano for you!" The process of building trust takes time. I kept sowing seeds as I saw opportunities to do so, showing her a vision of a future that she could enjoy.

One week I said, "You know, they're talking about discharge. I wonder what it would be like for you if we visited some places before you move?"

Surprisingly, she agreed, and we made a plan to visit a few assisted living facilities. From my experience, I anticipated that the facilities in the city would be unwilling to take her because of her history of behavioral issues. Even so, I took her to several at her request and filled out application paperwork. As I expected, none would accept her. Notably, while she was with me she never had a panic attack when leaving the hospital—it was her decision to go, and she had some things to potentially look forward to, so she didn't act out.

I decided to call a physician friend who owned some assisted living group homes in the suburbs. We talked at length about Carolyn's behavioral issues. Usually, she would not be an appropriate candidate for this type of group home because of the lack of oversight, but one of the homes had a piano and I really thought she could be calm there. I asked if my patient could be considered if I continued regular follow-up as a care manager.

The owner agreed. Carolyn visited the home and seemed to like it. Later, the home's activities coordinator came to the hospital to talk with her about living in the group home. They seemed to really get along with each other. Finally, Carolyn agreed to try out the group home.

I explained to her, "It will just be for a while until you decide if it is right for you. I want to make sure that wherever you are, you are comfortable." Again, all true. Although I certainly was hoping it would be a good fit for her, if she had hated it, I would have continued looking for other solutions. I made sure she had access to the piano and a phone right from the start, as we had talked about earlier. By being true to my word, I showed her again that her trust in me was well placed.

When the day finally came for her hospital discharge, I was the one transporting her to the new facility. I rolled her out in her wheelchair. As we passed by the nurses' station, she waved to them and said, "So long!"

They were all shocked! She had never acted like this before at discharge. Rather than showing any anxiety, she seemed excited about taking the next step.

She was genuinely ready to move on after she was exposed to little things that grew over time to help her make the decision. It started with going downstairs, then thinking about what it would be like to have a phone, then getting out and seeing some places that might work, and then meeting the activities coordinator. A lot of little nudges in the right direction helped her see this as a positive transition. I was careful not to direct her—I just volunteered the right kind of information at the right time. She made every decision along the way. And, importantly, she could still make a different decision down the road, since this was "just for a while until you decide what to do." I gave her agency, but also the information she needed to make good decisions that worked for everyone.

What a joy to see her happy in a new living situation! It meant so much to her that someone listened to her and took her seriously. Often, we overlook someone when they have a disability and we try to decide for them. As this story demonstrates, a person may become accepting of change if they are listened to and given time and patience and the right information. In the end, she adjusted well to the new facility and decided to stay.

A Specific Request

One woman's son, James, told me he lived with his elderly mother, but needed my help because she was not following her medication schedule. Also, she had some medical issues but did not want to go see her doctors. He told me that there was a dog in the house that was his mother's companion and was generally friendly.

I called her to let her know that her son had asked me to visit her as a backup in case he was unavailable. She agreed to a visit, but when I knocked on her door, she wouldn't open it. She said she had changed her mind. I could hear the dog barking loudly. I talked with her for a moment through the closed door and then agreed to leave.

A few days later, I returned and knocked on the door. She answered, keeping the door closed as before. This time I had a specific request. I knew she had been a nurse in her career and had written a book on nursing. I had found a copy of it and brought it with me to the visit. I told her

I returned because I had found the book she had written and was hopeful that she would sign the copy for me.

She grunted a bit, but let me in the house. She signed the book and then we talked for a few minutes about how she got into nursing. We had a good conversation, so I asked if I could return just once more so that she would know me better and could call me if she couldn't reach her son. She agreed.

The next visit, I asked if she had her medication delivered or had to have it picked up, and which pharmacy she used. She just seemed more relaxed and told me about her medications. She allowed me to measure her blood pressure and pulse. I told her that she had a really well-respected doctor and asked how long it had been since she had last visited her. She said, "Not in a long time but I don't really need to see her." "Okay," I replied. "Well, I'm sure you will visit her when you need your medications refilled." I thanked her for allowing my visit and told her that it really eased her son's mind knowing that we had met each other.

Regular visits continued after that point, which was such a relief. I enjoyed talking with her about nursing and was also able to assess her condition each time. I helped her solve a few other issues that were making her life more difficult than it needed to be. For example, she had difficulty getting out of a chair because it was too low, so when I informed her son James, he was able to find her a higher chair that was even more comfortable. She thanked him for switching it out.

Sometimes it's a very slow process to establish trust but it can happen even though there may be strong initial resistance.

———

Trust is fundamental to everything else you are trying to accomplish as a caregiver. Once your family member sees that something can work out positively with your assistance, they will have more faith in you because you have demonstrated that your words match your actions. That said, expect some bumps along the way. Some days it will be harder than others to gain your loved one's cooperation, but keep trying. With time and effort, relationship issues will be resolved, and you will notice that you are finally starting to work together as a team.

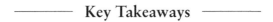

Key Takeaways

» Trust begins when you stay calm and look into your loved one's eyes.
» Trusting someone means that you believe them.
» If you want others to trust you, you need to trust them first.
» If your family member doubts you, they will work to hold on to control.
» Show them you are on their side by being nonjudgmental and encouraging.
» Your loved one can become accepting of change if you have patience and give them pertinent information.
» Allow time for relationship building.

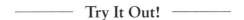

Try It Out!

Think of some ways you can show your family
member that you are on their side and try
them the next time you are with them.

CHAPTER SEVEN

ENCOURAGE INDEPENDENCE

Because it's so central to my approach, I've talked a lot in previous chapters about ways to determine our loved one's needs and how we can best care for them to maintain their health and happiness. Caregiving is a helping role but deciphering how to help can be a little tricky. Although patients' needs can change often, some ways of assisting are usually better for them than others.

Independence is about a person's ability to be self-reliant—to make their own decisions and to do for themselves. I believe in helping others maintain their abilities for as long as possible because it can lead to much more positive health outcomes. It's probably also been a priority for me with my patients because it's something I want for myself. I just love the feeling of independence! From what I've seen in my work, most people do. It makes us feel strong and capable, which is good for our self-esteem and overall health.

Helping our loved one function as normally as possible is the key to their autonomy. Even if they take a long time to button their shirt, for example, I allow them to do it if they can. I only intervene if they are truly unable to do it on their own. That is easier said than done because, as helpers, we don't want to see people struggle. Yet we know that some struggle in life has made us strong and independent. Let's offer that to the people we are caring for too.

Helping Too Much

Independence feels good to our patients, but it can also save the energy of caregivers. This is an important point, as our role takes so much of our energy, and it can lead to burnout. I'll talk about ways to prevent burnout in the final chapter of the book.

There are things that we do for others just to be kind, but we may be forgetting that allowing them to accomplish things on their own can actually be helpful to them. Even getting to do just part of a task can be meaningful and contribute to their sense of well-being.

Often when we visit our loved one, in an effort to get things done so we can quickly get back to our own responsibilities, we jump right in—cleaning their eyeglasses, folding their clothes, microwaving a meal for them, etc. We don't necessarily stop to think about whether they could be doing any of these things on their own.

Of course, many older people have limitations, but looking for what is still possible for them can quite literally extend their lives as they stay engaged and involved. It may take more time initially to work through what they can and can't do, or to look for adaptive ways for them to handle a particular task, but it can save you time in the long run.

Many studies have shown that older people can still learn, they just take longer to do it. Don't be discouraged if it takes your family member some time to master tasks. Patience is required.

For example, seniors can write emails if the computer is set up to make it easy for them. My mother taught herself to type in her eighties and wrote a weekly email to her seventeen grandchildren well into her nineties. She also started a knitting club and taught her friends at the senior residence to knit. Over the years they knitted hundreds of baby caps and donated them to the nursery at her local hospital. Engaging in volunteer efforts such as these can make seniors feel useful, which can bring great joy to them in their remaining years.

Older people may find it hard to remember too many steps, but their memory can be enhanced with visual cues. Once you have taught them a task, it can help to provide written instructions that they can refer to the next time they attempt it. Auditory cues can also be useful as reminders. People can often take their own meds, for example, when reminded by an alarm on their phone.

When we choose to help others when they can handle a task themselves, we are stealing that experience from them and hijacking an opportunity for them to apply their own energy to work through a life situation. Granted, it can be hard to watch someone strain a bit, but the outcome will bring them joy and a sense of accomplishment.

Transitions

Often once we've seen our loved one in the hospital, and have thought of them as "sick" or "injured," our desire to help them can cause us to jump in and take control. This arises from a good intention—we want to do everything we can to help keep them safe. The problem is that this adoption of a "sick role" while in the hospital can undermine the ability of people to act more autonomously once they get home.

The transition period can be an issue for both parties. We feel that we should be taking care of our loved one's every need, and become nervous about them being able to do what they used to. They become more vulnerable while in the hospital, which undermines their confidence. Once home, unsure of their skills and abilities, they may hesitate to resume many regular activities while they are recovering, pointing to the fact that they don't "feel ready" even as it becomes clear that they are capable.

The goal is to gradually move them from being a passive recipient of care to being more involved on every level, which is better for their self-esteem and overall well-being. It also tends to garner more cooperation from them as our confidence in them spurs their own. It's a delicate balance because capabilities can change from month to month. It's best to reevaluate their skills from time to time so you can adapt to their changing needs.

Verifying What They Can Do

If a patient tells me they are unable to do what they used to do, I don't immediately accept that as true until I verify it. Once they've had an injury or been in the hospital, some have told me that they can't walk or can never get a shower again or can't go out because they'd have to go down steps, etc. "They won't let me get them out of bed," some aides say. Checking the validity of the person's thoughts and always moving toward their highest potential results in much more happiness for them.

Again, we can turn to our motivational interviewing technique. Motivational interviewing suggests that there's a way to encourage people to move forward if we can figure out the necessary motivation rather than us imposing our will on them. That is always my goal with patients—to support change without directing them. The changes they make toward self-sufficiency will feel good to them in the end. I have seen this over and over.

Encouraging the Use of Adaptive Tools

Much of what we can do for our family members is to create the necessary conditions for autonomy. To figure out how our patients can do things safely. What adaptations to their environment and/or what pieces of equipment are necessary?

There are many adaptive measures that are useful when people are not able to manage on their own. Older people tend to balk at the idea of using equipment that is new to them, but once they try it and see that it is helpful, they often change their minds. I like to remind people that the eyeglasses most of us have been wearing since our forties are just tools to help us function better, and we don't give them a second thought. As our bodies age, we may need to start using additional tools, such as hearing aids, to help us remain independent.

Here is a list of some other useful devices:

» walkers
» canes
» risers for beds and chairs to make it easier to get in and out
» easy attach-and-remove handles to help them when getting in and out of cars
» poles for the bedside or toilet to hold onto when transferring
» handles in the bath or shower
» handrails for the bathroom
» elevated toilet seats
» smart watches
» devices with alarms that remind people to take their meds

You can locate most of these products by searching online for "durable medical equipment," which is a Medicare term for non-disposable medical products. The internet is a great source for finding items that can help a person feel independent. New adaptive devices are continually being invented.

I try to reinforce the idea that with some adaptation, aging adults can do so much more than they realize. Encouraging them to try will give meaning to their days and improve their quality of life. It's important to show them that you have faith in their abilities.

Initially, you will be involved with assisting your loved one until they become proficient with these devices, but often, with the right equipment, they can learn to perform the tasks on their own in a short period of time. They may want to give up at times, but once they find they can do things for themselves, they will begin to gain confidence both physically and emotionally.

Medical device companies can be of great assistance in this area, as can physical therapists and occupational therapists, who can evaluate what is needed. After a hospital stay, Medicare will often pay for physical and occupational therapy services for a limited period. Your loved one may be a bit resistant about having these professionals come to their home, especially if they have grown tired of having assessments, but I would encourage them to accept at least one visit from each specialty area, as the solutions they suggest can truly be life changing.

In addition to locating safety and ease-of-use devices and equipment for our loved ones, we can also help them organize their spaces to improve accessibility. Even organizing shelves by putting the most frequently used items in the front will be appreciated, especially if your loved one is visually impaired. Clearly labeling items using large print may help too.

My mother, who lived in an independent senior apartment, needed help twenty-four hours a day at one point. However, she didn't like the times that her aide was sitting nearby ready to help, but not actually busy at the moment. I bought an easy walkie-talkie for Mom (she did not use a cell phone), so that the aide could do laundry down the hall or sit on the sofa in the lobby near her apartment during slower moments. Mom learned how to call the aide to come help her to use the bathroom or for other needs. She appreciated having some alone time, and she no longer had to watch the aide "do nothing." Later, she wore a medical alert system that allowed her to talk directly into the device to contact assistance. The aide was also encouraged to invite Mom to do activities with her like play checkers or draw or paint or sew instead of waiting until she was needed.

Helping in the Background

As much as we like to be hopeful on behalf of our patients or loved ones, we must also be realistic. When people are truly not capable in certain areas, it's helpful to take care of those items for them. It should be done, though, without making much of a fuss about it. The idea is to encourage your loved one to do as much as they possibly can for themselves, but remain close and available should they need your assistance.

When we realize that they are no longer able to keep track of certain things on their own, that's when we need to help them in the background when possible. Occasionally, dates can be mixed up or forgotten and we can help by verifying with doctors' offices and checking to see if our loved one has the correct dates on their calendar. Doing this when you are not directly with them makes a difference because then they are not reminded of areas that are difficult for them. Your family member will still feel independent even if you are helping in the background, as long as you do it in an unobtrusive manner.

Making Medical Decisions

Making decisions about medical treatments is one area where it can be especially hard for caregivers to allow their loved ones to be autonomous. You may recall Margaret's story from Chapter 1. After discussing options with her doctor and carefully considering them, she decided that she didn't want any invasive end-of-life care and filled out the paperwork to confirm her choices. But when the time came, some family members questioned her decision. That debate is an example of how important it is to respect a person's wishes, even if—or perhaps especially if—you would have made a different choice.

When it comes to medical treatment, it's best for all members of the care team, including the patient, to work together cooperatively to evaluate available options.

Patient autonomy is defined in the medical community as the right of people to make decisions about their medical care without their health care provider or anyone else trying to unduly influence their decisions. Patient autonomy does allow for providers to educate the person, provide relevant research, and explain to them the pros and cons of any possible treatments. When people are encouraged to ask questions, list their concerns, and collaborate on treatment options, it improves the outcomes.

The following stories demonstrate various ways you can encourage your loved one to be self-sufficient:

That's Not Possible Anymore

Richard lived in an apartment with his wife. He had adequate finances for any medical care or medical devices that he needed. He was, however, very depressed from a recent stroke that limited his leg strength, and he was increasingly upset with this change.

He learned to be helped with a sponge bath in the bathroom, but he mentioned that in the past he had really enjoyed his showers. When I offered to help him take a shower, he told me, "That's not possible anymore." He had adapted to using a wheelchair and accepted being transferred, but he was not aware of equipment that could be used to assist him to take a shower. It all seemed too complicated to him. In one of my early visits, I touched on the topic of equipment, but he was too tired or depressed to take it in.

At the next visit I took a transfer shower chair with me. It's a seat that can slide across and lock over the tub to position someone for a shower. I purchased the equipment for my company to use for demonstration purposes. I had discovered during my career that sometimes actually seeing something in action is what patients will respond to, rather than just listening to someone describe equipment that could potentially help. He was the first to try it and I told him it was a demo unit. I explained that I needed to evaluate its helpfulness and ease of use, and asked him if he would tell me what it felt like to sit on it. I wanted to know if he would recommend it to others.

Something marvelous happened when I said that! While he may not have tried it just for himself, he was willing to try it out and provide feedback. Maybe he felt good that he was helping me as well as other future patients, which he was. For a man who had felt insignificant since his stroke, being able to help someone else seemed to energize him. Once he transferred onto the shower chair, I slid the chair over and lifted his legs so that everything was in the tub and aligned for a shower. The seat locked in place, which helped him feel secure. He accepted having an aide assist him with a shower, and he helped by washing anywhere he could manage.

Remember: a person feels healthier when they do as much as possible on their own. It may take longer, but it feels better and can even help improve their physical strength. Prior to this day, Richard just passively allowed someone to sponge bathe him without his active participation.

He seemed upbeat and renewed after his shower. I thanked him genuinely for describing what it felt like to him and what things made the event easier for him.

It's so helpful to question it when someone says that they are unable to do something. After this experience, Richard was able to take a shower regularly and it improved his mood and feeling of independence.

I Don't Think I Can

My strong belief is that it is important to help everyone return to as much normalcy as possible after an illness or injury. Or, more accurately, to return to whatever their particular version of "normal" looks like. This seems to encourage them and improve their outlook on life.

One of my patients, Brian, was transferred to a group home after a full year in a nursing home. His wife lived in the same group home, and they were very happy to finally be together again. Brian had not been out of bed for over a year due to back pains. They eventually were relieved, but because he had needed the bedrest for so long, bedrest had become a habit for him and the staff, rather than a necessity.

Soon after his arrival at the group home, he told me that he was sad to have to stay in bed all the time. I asked his physician if I could try to get him up, and he agreed. I then asked Brian what he thought of trying some time out of bed. He said, "I don't think I can."

I answered, "Maybe not, but let's approach it very slowly and see what you can do."

He started with sitting and dangling his legs over the side of the bed. I sat next to him to physically support him. He felt dizzy and unstable at first, but gradually he built up his tolerance so that he became comfortable sitting alone on the side of the bed.

Before long, he agreed to try a transfer into a wheelchair. He liked it but mentioned that he got tired easily. I always listened and responded to his need to return to bed when he requested it.

He had a bit of foot drop (difficulty lifting the front part of his foot) as a result of lying in bed without enough ankle support. His physician agreed to have a physical therapist help him with strengthening exercises. It took a full year, but eventually he was able to walk again, slowly, with a walker. He still used the wheelchair for longer distances but was able to use the walker when he could. It was just an amazing effort on his part.

What a journey for him to go from being confined to his bed to being able to walk out to the porch of the group home and sit there with his wife! It certainly required patience and effort on his part, but he was highly motivated.

His smile was huge when he was with others, and he became friends with everyone in the facility. I think having respect for all humans allows us to want the best for them. The ability to be mobile—if at all possible—allows one's world to open up and a feeling of normalcy to emerge. My motto is "It's always worth a try."

If Brian had not been able to tolerate the wheelchair, a lounge chair might have been an alternative for him so he could be more upright and out of bed. I always ask what precisely is keeping a patient in bed or in a wheelchair. There are many times when it is necessary, but sometimes it's just because that's how they ended up after a medical event and no one ever nudged them to go further.

I recommend taking the initiative to help the medical staff become more aware of your loved one's previous abilities so that their therapy will be directed toward returning to that level as they recover.

He Had No Right

A new client, Michael, called to tell me that he had just brought his parents back to Maryland from Florida, where they lived in the winter. Evidently a concerned neighbor in Florida had reported to him that some of his parents' behavior was unusual. They noticed some forgetfulness and trouble with decision-making. This was all unexpected for the son, and he quickly flew to his parents' winter home to bring them back to their summertime condo, which was near his house. He seemed panicked because both parents were angry with him for cutting short their time in the warm weather.

Michael asked if I could come over right away to help him sort things out. He did not want to leave his parents in their condo in this agitated state, but he had to return to his own family. I agreed to make a visit within the hour.

I went over to help ease the situation for all involved. When I arrived, his parents were not speaking to Michael and did not want me to be there. His mother, Annie, said, "He had no right to call you." Then both parents began yelling at him. Annie was ready to call the train station to book a ticket for them both to return to Florida.

I said, "Oh, this seems like a difficult evening for you, and you must be so tired from your trip."

They agreed. Then I said, "Let me think this through with each of you one at a time so we don't all talk at once."

Annie agreed to speak with me alone in the kitchen while Michael and her husband, David, talked things over in the living room. That gave us some private time for her to be fully heard.

She explained that she had been taking good care of David since he had some memory loss, and her son was just "being mean." She said that Michael wanted them to have twenty-four-hour care now, which was unnecessary as she was her husband's caregiver. I told her that my role was to help Michael understand that his dad could be made safe, which would ease some of the tension.

I asked Annie to tell me everything about the situation so that I could understand what would have caused her neighbor to be so concerned. I also asked what tasks were involved in David's care. She did not have an explanation for why the neighbor would tell Michael they were concerned. She began listing David's care needs. She told me that she filled his medication box weekly, and I said that medications were a good place to start.

I asked for his medication list so that I could see what he was taking each day. She didn't have one and was not quite sure of all the medications, which was a big red flag for me. She mainly took a pill out of each medication container each day to give to him. I told her that Michael would likely relax if we showed him exactly how his father's care is organized. I offered to help her gather the prescription information so that we could give Michael a copy in writing. It seemed to ease her mind that there might be a way to help him understand.

I wrote down David's medications—or at least as much as Annie could remember—and asked if we could confirm the list with his doctor the next day. That way, Michael would trust the medications since they were verified. Annie and I made a plan to fill the organizer together the next day, including having her put the actual pills in the correct slot according to what was listed on the verified form. That allowed her to maintain a measure of control and still feel that she was her husband's primary caretaker.

I told her I would type out the list and bring it with me the next morning. I explained that it would help me if there was ever a time that she was not there to fill the pill box herself. Although she had some memory loss too, I never mentioned it to her as a potential issue. That would come later. My sense was that she needed to continue to feel in control. After our conversation, we returned to the living room to present our proposal. All seemed to agree, and things were momentarily calm. I visited the next day and followed up on our plan.

I found both Annie and David to be quite charming and intelligent. They had been well respected in their community throughout their lives. Despite memory issues, both could hold a normal conversation for the most part and seemed to relax as we chatted about many different topics. My love of people and their life stories allowed me to easily relate to them both.

Initially, my goal was to gently guide Annie in documenting her husband's needs. David did not seem to care that they were pulled away from Florida, except that he did not want his wife to be upset. Although he seemed to know that his memory was diminishing, he didn't see it as a major issue. I sensed that he would go along with anything that Annie thought was good for them both.

Annie then shared that David was not very thorough when he showered (for example, he would forget to wash his hair) and that she was always afraid he might fall. There were no handrails in the bathroom shower for him to hold on to. She agreed to safety bars to ease her concern.

I asked David if I could assess his needs while he showered to make sure he was safe. He agreed, which surprised me, so I went early the next morning to do the assessment. I told him that I would like to hand him the liquid soap and shampoo containers when he needed them so that he didn't have to reach to the floor to pick them up. (I noted that we should install a shelf to hold them so that it would be easier for him in the future.) To help him stay on track, I said, "I have the shampoo right here for you to use when you are done washing your face." This phrasing allowed me to remind him to wash both his face and hair instead of directing him to do so. The wording we use is so important to promote autonomy. He then allowed me to wash his back and legs, as he seemed to lose balance when leaning over. In the end, I wanted him to feel that he took his own shower, even though I was there assisting and guiding him.

Over time, the couple adapted to living in the north without their winter trips to Florida. Early on I visited often, but later they accepted an aide who drove them where they needed to go, including to doctor visits, out to dinner, etc. That was so fun for them! I was happy that they became so comfortable with the aide, who they thought of as their "friend." I continued my oversight, attended their physician visits, and helped with problem-solving when necessary. Their son Michael felt such relief.

Helping "in the background" allows our loved one to feel so much more independent. As caregivers, we need to nurture that independence as it gives the person a sense of normalcy, something we all desire.

We Can Do It for Her

When I met my patient Hilda, she lived alone in an apartment building. The building's laundry machines were on a different floor from her, so she had a neighbor do the wash for her. On one visit when I thought she was ready to do more on her own, I asked her to help me do the laundry.

She responded, "I can't." I encouraged her just to try it with me to see how it felt for her. She agreed to try, and soon we were doing the laundry together. She began to realize that she had not lost all her capabilities to do things on her own. She did have to deal with the uncertainty and doubt she felt—she was often hesitant—but by working with me she was able to handle it.

Eventually she moved to an assisted living facility. One day when visiting her, I noticed that an aide brought freshly washed and folded clothes into her room. I asked her if Hilda was permitted to do her own laundry with my help. She said, "Oh, we can do it for her." I said, "I know you can, but she and I can do it if we're allowed to use the machines." The aide agreed, so Hilda and I began doing her laundry together again. I didn't want her to lose any of her skills since she was indeed capable of doing more and more on her own. Doing tasks together is a great interim step. By observing us, our loved ones can see exactly how to perform a task, and eventually they may be able to do more of it on their own.

The aides recognized our goal of achieving as much independence for Hilda as possible and were very cooperative about it. They began accompanying her to the washer and dryer rather than just doing the laundry themselves. I was hopeful that at some point she could perform the task independently, but that would take some time. With the aides' help, Hilda was able to practice regularly with supervision, which was a very helpful step in her path toward independence.

Occasionally it's a nice treat for someone to do something for us that we can do for ourselves, but independence should always be encouraged as much as possible. It helps us feel good about ourselves by giving us a sense of accomplishment. Aging adults often lose their sense of being useful unless there is a helpful activity that they can manage to do on their own. I have observed many patients giving up on tasks too easily because they no longer feel competent, but it's likely they could be accomplishing many of them with some encouragement and assistance.

———————

Helping others feel as autonomous as possible is a great gift to them that brings both pleasure and a sense of purpose to their lives. Although seniors may regress in some areas, they are still adults. Our parents, especially, still want to feel like our parents. As I've mentioned, when we act as though we are in charge of them, it likely will cause them to feel rebellious. When we look to them to make their own choices, it helps them relax and think more clearly.

Always acknowledge their accomplishments and involve them in solutions whenever possible. Allowing your loved one to take care of as much as they are capable of on their own, even if it takes some oversight, gives them strength. It's good for them to have agency over their own lives to the extent possible. Their feeling of independence and purpose is critical to maintaining good mental health. No matter what stage of life we're in, it's healthy for all of us to remain as autonomous as possible.

——————— **Key Takeaways** ———————

» Independence can lead to much more positive health outcomes.

» Know that it is natural to want to help with everything, but helping is only beneficial if the help is really needed.

» Don't accept what you've heard about a loved one's abilities without verifying its validity. Remember that it's always worth a try!

» Only intervene if a person is truly unable to accomplish a task on their own, even if it is taking them a long time.

» Your loved one can still feel independent if someone is "helping in the background," as long as the help is provided in an unobtrusive manner.

» Explore the many adaptive tools and devices that can help your family member do a task on their own.

» Keep encouraging them to move forward so they can reach their maximum potential.

——————— **Try It Out!** ———————

Look for a task your loved one is likely to be
able to perform on their own or with minimal
help and encourage them to try it. Notice how
they feel after accomplishing that task.

CHAPTER EIGHT

BE PATIENT

Throughout this book, I've shared various aspects of my approach with you. My hope is that as you consider each of these concepts and begin to integrate them into your caregiving process, your frustration level will decrease. This will help you to be more tolerant of your loved one even when they are needy or noncompliant.

Of all the tools I've mentioned so far, patience may be the most important one for caregivers.

When I was still a child, my grandmother told me that I was very patient. It just seemed to be natural for me, and I loved that she noticed it about me. While I had many internal fears and anxieties as a young person, I never doubted that displaying outer calmness was just part of my personality. It was an innate gift, and I will forever be thankful that it led me to my life's work.

I was taught in my nursing program that patience is "the capacity to accept or tolerate delay, trouble, or suffering without becoming angry or upset." My training helped to further develop this capacity as I learned to be more empathetic toward my patients and what they were going through. Over the course of my career, I developed more skills and techniques that allowed me to head off many conflicts with others.

Patience and empathy may come more naturally to some than others, but I feel strongly that every single person can be a peacemaker, especially with those you love or care for. It's something that each of us can practice more and more each day so that it becomes a habit.

Patience is a skill that can be honed over time. Having the right mentality built on empathy and respect for the other person makes it easier to be patient with them. It is a strategy for harmony in our relationships that is worth striving for, even though it can be challenging in the heat of the moment.

As an example, imagine you are driving and someone cuts you off and speeds away. Your initial reaction might be to feel anger and frustration—how dare they? But if you knew that the person in the car was driving someone to the hospital because of a medical emergency, you would understand their actions a bit better and be able to forgive them. Understanding the reason or rationale behind an action really changes our ability to be patient with others. This chapter is intended to give you many alternative explanations for behaviors you might normally consider to be frustrating. Once you understand some of the underlying causes for why a person might be being "difficult" on a given day, it becomes easier to be patient with them.

Understanding What Can Affect Your Loved One's Personality

In previous chapters I've mentioned some of the ways that loved ones in our care can be difficult for us. As you can see from the following list, aging bodies and psyches, along with growing medical issues, can significantly impact how family members in our care interact with us.

Issues that can make seniors less cooperative:

» They may be in pain or discomfort.
» They generally have lower energy, making them less likely to want to do things.
» Their senses are diminished so things don't look right, smell right, or taste right to them, or are too hot or too cold. They can't see or hear as well, which is frustrating for them.

» They may have memory loss, especially short-term memory.
» It often takes them longer to learn new information, and they don't retain it as well.
» They are increasingly emotional and vulnerable, more easily frustrated, and more anxious.

These issues can result in the following behaviors:
» They may be more tied to their routines, which make them feel comfortable, and resistant to any changes.
» They may have a tendency to exaggerate or diminish medical issues.
» They are often more repetitive in their conversations, excessively worrying about or "looping" on various topics.
» They can be more needy, wanting more of our time than we're able to give.
» They can be less sensitive to others and their needs, which can feel dismissive.

Even some who have always been reasonable and easy to deal with in the past can change when health issues arise. As their fears and frustrations increase, they can become more challenging to be with. They may become demanding, overly dependent, or full of anxiety. They can begin to act out in ways you haven't seen before. They might withdraw, call out to you constantly, or become belligerent. Since this has not been their normal behavior, it can be confusing and even scary to witness these changes.

Others who were already difficult may become even more extreme. They may become whiny, bossy, paranoid, or overly concerned about safety or money. Be sure to communicate any of these changes in their personalities to their doctors. They may be related to a new condition or may be a side effect of a medication. Often some of these situations can be treated or corrected, but it may take time.

I often hear the following from family members who are caring for their loved ones:

- » "She just keeps complaining. I can't take it anymore."
- » "He keeps repeating over and over and over. It grates on my nerves."
- » "He just keeps forgetting. It's hard to watch."
- » "She won't cooperate. It doesn't matter what I say."
- » "She keeps changing her mind, which takes up extra time on my part to work out the issue."
- » "He is so unsafe but won't accept any changes. It's just so frustrating."
- » "His poor decisions affect me because I have to work to correct things."
- » "She keeps wanting me out of her business but there is no one else to help her. I am feeling more and more angry about this."
- » "Her anger is infuriating. I can't listen to it anymore."
- » "He keeps criticizing all that I do. It's demeaning but he needs my help."
- » "He won't spend his money for services but he really needs them now."
- » "He is not safe at home alone but doesn't accept that. It's a constant worry for me."

Each of these situations represent a legitimate problem to face. I have had similar thoughts myself and always have to think through the best way to manage my interactions to keep myself calm and focused.

It can be so difficult to see these changes and try to figure out how to be helpful without becoming overly anxious yourself. Your loved one may be responding out of fear or pain or lack of control. This is understandable, but it creates difficult interactions nonetheless. As family members, our own fears and anxieties about their condition may come into play as well, which can limit our ability to be calm and comforting to them.

Below are some ideas for developing a patient mindset, coping with your loved one when they are not at their best, and handling your own frustrations. These protective measures will help you have a better caregiving experience.

Developing a Patient Mindset

Remember your goal. At different stages of our lives, we have needed others to be patient with us and our behavior. Our parents certainly had to be tolerant when we were teenagers and were not cooperative or were making poor choices. One thing that helps me to be tolerant when I get frustrated is to remember my goal of maintaining a good relationship with my patient. I can then use the strength of our connection, and the bond between us, to obtain more cooperation so that I can provide them the best possible care.

Tap into your own experience. No matter our age, it can take time for us to make changes even when we're motivated to make them. When others are patient and tolerant with us, we feel well loved. When they give us their time and attention, when they listen to us and offer advice that's in our best interest as we are going through transitions, we really appreciate it. When we are able to be similarly patient with others and achieve a good outcome as a result, it reminds us how important our own role is in our interactions.

Practice acceptance. Sometimes, despite our desire to remain close, we have to accept that difficult loved ones are not likely to change, especially if they are getting on in age. This can be incredibly hard to do and it may take some time to process. But once you accept it and grieve the loss, you can begin to take steps to make the best of the relationship as it is now. Changing your own behavior by breaking out of toxic cycles is often the only thing that can improve these relationships. It might surprise you how well this works in practice. You cannot directly control someone else's behavior, but you can control your reactions to it. Your calm, patient communication can have a positive influence on their behavior as well!

Tips for Coping with Your Family Member When They Are Not Cooperating

Try not to argue. Most of us have a natural tendency to try to defend our position when we feel attacked or questioned. Some personalities go further and truly enjoy arguing, or "getting under your skin," for its own sake. They will put you on the defensive and try to pull you into the argument because it is a kind of game to them. It's important to break out of the reactive cycle, which only maintains your suffering and yields them more attention. First, you need to identify what you want or need yourself before entering into a conversation with them. Otherwise, they may begin to argue with you before you've had a chance to think through the best solution. Try to present a calm and gentle demeanor as you tell them what works for you, and then end the discussion if need be. We often think that arguing will convince someone to try "our" way, but it usually leads nowhere.

Become curious. Rather than respond in an argumentative way, try being curious. Instead of telling them what to do, ask what they need or want. This lets them know that you care about them and are on their side. Consider saying "I'm trying to understand what makes this so important to you." So often people will say they don't like the food and their well-meaning relative or caregiver will say, "…but you have to eat!" Sometimes there is a simple solution that we are not aware of. Maybe they want the food to be warmer or cooler or softer. Finding out that information is a start to problem-solving.

Reference medical orders. Sometimes uncooperative patients will find suggestions and reminders more palatable if they come from someone other than a family member. Try using the language "Your doctor would like you to cut down on sugar" or "Your physical therapist wants you to do your exercises three times a week" to see if that helps with compliance.

Tips for Handling Your Frustration

Step away. When you feel yourself getting heated, step away from the conversation. Excuse yourself to go to the restroom if needed. Even a momentary break can help you cool down and reconsider how you should handle things. Taking a few deep breaths can make you feel calmer. Stepping away can allow you to get in touch with your empathy again. Then you can try to be more aware of the impact of your words and actions and their ripple effect on your loved one. Pulling back from our anger and frustration and instead becoming curious again about the behaviors of others takes the pressure off them and us as well. They will be more likely to see us as a source of support—as someone on the same team.

Don't force the issue. Sometimes you just need to wait and try again another day. Perhaps it would go better if you let someone else try. Forcing the issue is never the right answer, even if what you are trying to accomplish is for the good of the person you are caring for. If you do lose your cool, try to be kind to yourself. We are all imperfect humans. Just regroup and try again to move forward when the time is right.

Don't enable. When faced with strong or angry personalities, it's tempting to walk on eggshells or tiptoe around them. As much as possible, resist the urge to do so, as it can lead to a lot of distress. Behave as normally as you can around them. Calmly let them know what you can and cannot do. When pressured to do something you don't want to do, try saying "that's not going to work for me today" rather than giving a specific excuse that they can then argue against. Learn not to take in hurtful words from them. Try saying "Oh, my goodness, that felt hurtful," to let them know the impact of their unkind words, and then let it go so it doesn't ruin your day. Disengage if the discussion gets heated, because anger will not solve the issue.

Establishing Healthy Boundaries

One reason many family caregivers experience frustration in their role is because of weak or nonexistent boundaries. If you are a people-pleaser, especially when it comes to family members, it may create a lot of hardship for you. There is a lot of good information on the internet and many helpful books that discuss how to develop boundaries. I highly recommend *The Book of Boundaries: Set the Limits That Will Set You Free* by Melissa Urban. It is well worth your while to learn what boundaries are, why they are critical for healthy relationships, and how to communicate them respectfully but assertively. There are also strategies for dealing with resistance to them. It is important to pay attention to your loved one's needs, but it's equally important to honor your own needs. You will learn more about this concept in Chapter 12.

The story below will give you an idea of the type of frustrating events you may encounter and how staying calm can allow you to work toward a solution:

Give Me Your Spiel and Leave!

One time a man named Jerry called me to say that his mom, Anita, was on continuous oxygen and needed help in the home but did not want to accept anyone. Once I explained to him ways that I could help her, Jerry hired me to see if she would respond and accept assistance.

At the first visit, I went to the door and knocked. Anita cracked open the door a tiny bit and held her cane up as though she were ready to hit me with it if I tried anything funny. With a bit of a scowl, she laid it out: "My son said you were coming. Just give me your spiel and leave."

It was not the best way to be greeted, but I took it in stride by telling myself that maybe she was afraid of me or afraid of change or just wanted to be left alone.

Undaunted, I said, "May I come in just for a few moments to explain what I do?" She sighed heavily and said, "Hurry up!" I went in and said, "I'm only going to take ten minutes and then I'm leaving." Anita reluctantly agreed.

Once inside, I didn't jump right into my talk, which I assumed would be met with similar animosity. Instead, I drew on what I knew about her and said, "I know you used to have a business, and I have a small business. At some time in the future, I would love to ask you a few questions about how you ran your business and see if you have any ideas that could work for me, since you have a lot more experience than I do."

She became excited and started to talk all about her business. After a few minutes, I said, "Now I'm only here for a few minutes so I guess I better give you my spiel and leave." I began to let her know all the things a care manager could do for her. After a bit I stopped and said, "Well, it's been ten minutes, so I guess I better leave." Anita said it was fine for me to be there, and that I could stay since we were just chatting.

I stuck to my promise and left anyway but said that it would be nice to talk with her again. From that point forward, I didn't have any problem with Anita inviting me into her home. Gradually, over several months, she began to really trust me.

Since I had met her, I had noticed that her personal hygiene was not being taken care of properly. It was obvious that she was not showering, changing clothes, or taking care of her fingernails at all. The house itself was also quite a mess and clearly had not been cleaned in ages. Recognizing her resistance to care, I started small and tried to do her fingernails, which were quite dirty and untrimmed. I said to her, "My daughter gave me a gift card once to get my nails done and I didn't really want to go because it was unfamiliar to me. When I finally accepted the offer, I was amazed at how soothing it felt." She said, "Well, I have no need for that."

I excused myself and went to her bathroom. I found a small bowl and filled it with warm, soapy water. With a towel over my shoulder, I returned to her and knelt in front of her. "What are you doing?" she said. I said, "I would just love to give you the same incredible feeling that I had when my hands were washed and rubbed with lotion."

She gave me a disgruntled look but put her hand in the water. I was so pleased with her reaction! I really thought she would put up more of a fight. We talked for a while, and I swished the water over her hand. Then she said, "Well, that's enough." I eased her hand out of the water, dried it off, and applied lotion.

She was talking the whole time as I did this, so I began trimming her nails as well. When I was done, she again said that she'd had enough.

We finished and she looked at me and smiled. I knew that the other hand would have to wait for another day but was pleased with my progress.

Many people in this same scenario may have pushed hard to get that second hand done, but I allow things to progress slowly as long as there is progress. Pushing too hard can lead to setbacks and more resistance. Even for me, this visit required extreme patience because it was so hard for me to leave with the many problems I knew could be fixed—one unwashed hand with untrimmed fingernails, a bit of a smell to her, and unkempt hair. I wished I could have taken care of everything and shown her how nice it felt to be clean and fresh, but I had to take my small accomplishment and hope to build on it in the future.

Very gradually, she allowed me to give her a shower, wash her hair, and regularly change her clothes. I found her an aide who also was a hairdresser who began doing her hair weekly. Over time Anita trusted the aide more and more so that she was then able to provide more personal care for Anita and also clean up the house.

She still would not allow a carpet cleaning company to come, so I took a small carpet cleaner (that looked like a vacuum) with me and cleaned a small area on each visit without resistance from her. Eventually she and her apartment smelled clean, and on Christmas day her son picked her up to have dinner with his family and was ecstatic that she looked and smelled good and seemed so calm and happy.

Moving slowly and steadily can pay off over time, even if it seems like it's not going to change things. One small step at a time can get you there eventually. Without the trust I established with her, and the patience I showed her, none of the rest of it could have happened.

I often wonder what I will be like for my children when some malady interferes with my quality of life. Hopefully, I will remember my own experience with my patients who exhibited difficult behaviors and will make their job as easy as I can. Still, no caregiving role is easy.

Keep in mind that you may have a lot of missteps as you are learning to put the tips in this chapter into practice. But as you become more confident, your frustration and feelings of helplessness will begin to decrease.

―――――― **Key Takeaways** ――――――

» Communicate any marked personality changes in your loved one to their doctor.
» Remember that they may be responding out of fear or pain or lack of control. Understanding these underlying reasons can help you be more patient with them.
» Try not to argue. Learn to become curious instead.
» Slow steps still represent progress. Keep trying to move forward together.
» Accept that your loved one may not be able to change.
» Establish healthy boundaries. Learn to communicate respectfully but assertively.
» If you feel yourself getting heated, step away from the conversation temporarily.
» Learn to expect frequent changes in your family member's moods and behaviors so that you can remain calm.
» Try doing what you don't want (changing your own behavior) in order to achieve what you do want (a better outcome).

―――――― **Try It Out!** ――――――

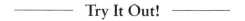

Pay attention to the times when you tend to get
frustrated. See if you can come up with new
ways of viewing situations or some calming
statements to get you through those moments
when you are feeling very impatient.

CHAPTER NINE

BE FLEXIBLE

Because a patient or loved one's condition can change from day to day, our work as caregivers can as well. No two days are the same, and we need to have a mindset that allows us to handle changes with grace. Being flexible—having the willingness to change or compromise, often on a dime—is a hard concept for those of us who feel better with a plan and a schedule. Plans are a positive thing and have their time and place, but if we are too rigid, it can set up a conflict that will make our work even more difficult.

Like acceptance, patience, and empathy, flexibility is another one of those attributes that may not come easily to you in your role. When you are caring for your loved one, there is so much to be done within a limited time frame. It's easy for caregivers to get overwhelmed by the enormity of all there is to do for the person we're caring for. It can help to set just a few simple goals for each visit, while still being open to and leaving some time for new issues that may have cropped up since the last time you saw them.

Any change in the plan, however small, can be frustrating if it keeps you from accomplishing your goals. It can be tempting to insist on doing things your way just to get the job done. My advice to you is to try to resist that temptation. In this chapter I will explain why it's so important to be flexible, and how there is another path that encourages cooperation rather than stifles it.

Expecting the Unexpected

Changing conditions come with the territory of caregiving more than in other areas of our lives. It's just a reality. Life sometimes surprises us, and things can change in the blink of an eye. When plans go awry, it throws us off balance. We may be temporarily shocked, and perhaps angry or saddened if there's a disappointment involved—and then ultimately resigned as we realize that we will have to adjust to the new reality.

When our patient or loved one's health takes a sudden turn or their needs change dramatically, we may feel more challenged than usual. You may think you are stopping by for a quick check on your loved one before going out for the evening, only to find they are lying on the floor from a fall, or they're having a bathroom emergency, or their skin is too warm to the touch. You will need to assess things quickly and make a new plan, which may involve calling for backup, taking them to see a doctor, or even calling 911.

Note: Most of the time, utilizing the rescue squad is the safest way to transport a person to the hospital. It allows them to be quickly taken directly to the emergency room to be seen. Also, a medical assessment will be done prior to the transport. Sometimes it is determined that it's possible for the person to be safely treated at home. If we choose to drive them ourselves and a crisis occurs on the way, we may not be prepared to take care of it.

However badly we may feel for our loved one, our first thought when these crises occur is often for ourselves: we don't have the time to deal with *one more difficult thing*! These are the moments when it is tough to be flexible, but we have no choice except to stop what we were doing, evaluate the situation, and figure out what's needed.

Adjusting Your Perspective

I've discussed in previous chapters the reasons our aging or ill loved ones may not be as cooperative as we'd like on a good day, let alone during an upsetting event. Think of how you feel when you are sick. You may not want to shower or eat. You may want to stay in bed all day. You may be more cranky or testy and want to do things your own way more than usual. Your family member is no different, except that their situation may be more chronic, whereas yours is likely to be short-lived. They may also have memory issues or daily pain that may exacerbate the situation.

It is challenging to stay calm when you feel like screaming, but there are steps you can take to help you stay levelheaded. Most of them have to do with changing your perspective, and avoiding *catastrophizing*, which is the tendency to think of the worst possible outcome of any situation. Whether the challenges are big or small, most things can be resolved, and hopefully some of the ideas in this chapter will help you manage your emotions so you can think clearly and make good decisions as you are working through the issues.

Understanding Why You Have to Be the Flexible One

In general, we like all our relationships to be fair and balanced, with a natural give and take. As young people, we learn to be gracious and somewhat deferential—to consider others' needs and to take turns, and we expect others to do the same for us.

In certain types of relationships, however, there is an inherent unfairness, and this can be hard to adjust to, especially if you are new to your role. In helping relationships like caregiving, because of their compromised health, patients need more consideration than their caregivers. This is true for all healthcare professionals, especially therapists and counselors. There is no getting around it—these relationships are always somewhat imbalanced.

This is where professional caregivers probably have an advantage, as they are not looking for love and concern from their patients the way adult children or other relatives are. (As I've mentioned, in Chapter 12

I suggest ways for you to get support and replenish your energy so that you can continue to offer this type of emotional support to your loved one.)

In my role as a care manager, as I was mediating between adult children and their aging parents, I often encountered questions similar to these: "Why should *we* have to be flexible instead of expecting our parents to be?" and "Why can't *they* just do what we need them to do?"

The answer is that as people age, they naturally become more rigid, often due to increasing anxiety. Their routines sustain them by providing predictability. Changes are upsetting to them, and it's hard for them to adapt. Seniors also get embarrassed more easily, especially when they need our help after being self-sufficient their whole lives.

Being younger, physically stronger, and more psychologically resilient, we are the ones who can more easily adapt. Aging adults in our care need *us* to be accepting of changes in their feelings, behaviors, and their health. This is not to say that we should allow ourselves to be abused or be taken advantage of. Rather, we must be the ones to set the example for healthy interactions.

Author Gary Zukav suggests in *The Seat of the Soul* that we may often have to be the ones to "go first" in our relationships to show others the way. As he explains, "If our actions create harmony and empowerment in another, we also will come to feel that harmony and empowerment." In other words, when we make an effort to be flexible, our patients or loved ones will sense that we are trying to adapt to their needs and may respond in kind.

Hopefully, at least on their better days, they will also be concerned about our well-being. Most of our loved ones do not actually want to be a burden. Know that they often feel grateful even if they don't express it to you often.

Expanding Your Capacity

It's important to learn what to do when our loved one's situation throws us for a loop. Instead of approaching it from a fearful, irritated stance, we can work on expanding our capacity to handle change when it happens. As I've mentioned before, we need to challenge our own thinking that our way (or what we see as the most efficient way) is the best. This sets up a power struggle that can damage the relationship and reduce our ability to help.

Rather than being overly tied to a certain outcome, we can remain open to possibilities we had not considered. You don't have to ignore your frustration if something doesn't go your way. Just make the decision to move beyond it after you acknowledge it to yourself. Let it be there but keep going and figure out another way.

Being flexible and adaptable is not so much about changing your mind or giving in as it is about allowing yourself to adapt to an ever-changing environment to accomplish your loved one's goals as well as your own tasks. Life constantly throws us curveballs. Research shows that people who are flexible tend to be some of the happiest and most successful in life and at work. Although it may take practice, it will be worth your while to try to expand your capacity to adapt. Don't we all prefer interacting with easygoing people?

Tips for Becoming More Flexible

» Relax your mind so it can stretch. Think of it as a rubber band.
» Ask yourself: "What's the worst that could happen if something doesn't go the way I want it to?"
» Be honest with yourself. Is what your family member wants *really* not okay, or is it just not the way you originally envisioned it?
» Use your imagination to come up with multiple options for every problem. What is the deeper goal the task is meant to achieve, and are there other ways of accomplishing it?

Dealing With Difficult Behaviors

A decade ago, I attended a talk for nursing staff and the presenter asked us, "How many people are dealing with someone who is difficult for them?" Not surprisingly, everyone raised their hands.

Then she asked, "How many of *you* are difficult to deal with?"

Not a single hand went up, but there were a few uncomfortable chuckles as people realized the implication of what they had been asked. It was such a short interaction, but I've always remembered it because it raised my awareness about how easy it is to get frustrated with *others*, but how none of us like to think that *we* are difficult. We may not be aware of ever being wrong or difficult to deal with, but obviously we must be at some times to some people. Even when we treat people the way we would want to be treated, some may find that our words or actions make us hard to deal with. It is critical to recognize this, as it opens the door to think of different ways to interact with others.

You may have to do some emotional work to deal with the unfairness of you being the one who needs to change, but this will be very good practice for all of your relationships. This balance of power issue is explored in depth in a book titled *Conscious Communication: How to Establish Healthy Relationships and Resolve Conflict Peacefully while Maintaining Independence* by Miles Sherts, which I recommend.

At some point, each of us will be thought of as difficult by someone we interact with; this is because we are all different from one another. Being perceived as difficult by someone else isn't a personality flaw; it's just that certain actions or mannerisms or ways of speaking or thinking can come across as "difficult" to other people and make them not want to deal with us. The more extreme the difference, the more we may seem challenging to other people. It helps me to recognize this so I can be more patient with others and try to adapt to make conversations and interactions easier.

Keeping an open mind regarding how we affect others also helps us to be more flexible for better results. Our self-talk can change from "she thinks I am being difficult," to "something I am doing is bothering her. I need to find out what that is so that we can better communicate."

Using De-escalation Techniques

De-escalation is a technique that can be used when your family member becomes increasingly upset with you or a situation at hand. For example, one of my patients once got so upset that I was leaving after a visit that she stood in front of my car, screaming at me. I went up to her and said, "You're having a stressful day. What if I sit with you for five more minutes until you are more ready to say goodbye for today?" She agreed, and it worked.

The term de-escalation involves transferring your sense of calm to another person so that you can have a more reasonable discussion. This is accomplished by: 1) showing genuine interest in what the person wants to tell you, 2) being nonjudgmental about what you hear, and 3) showing them empathy for what they are going through. These actions can defuse the strong emotion the person is feeling, returning them to a state where they are better able to listen to you.

In addition, it can help to give them some personal space when they are agitated. I've mentioned that I sometimes "make myself busy," doing a small task that needs to be done in the room, or even excusing myself to use the restroom, just to move away from a patient and disengage from the conversation for a few minutes. The goal is to stay calm yourself, rather than overreacting.

It can help to ignore others' more aggressive or challenging questions, which are likely just attention-getters (or attempts to "get under your skin" as I mentioned in the last chapter). Some people like to lash out when they are upset. It is important to set limits so that you are not abused—I don't tolerate patients screaming at me or threatening me. Walk away briefly, if necessary, but communicate that you want to have a calm conversation with them on your return. It's okay to tell them you need a minute to think. Ideally you can figure out a solution that will work for both of you.

It's also important to give your patient or loved one time to calm themselves down, regroup, and to begin to think more clearly. If there's a decision that needs to be made, try not to press them. Let them know that they can take some time to consider the issue at hand. Important decisions can require multiple discussions as together you weigh the pros and cons and explore options.

Keep in mind that when you first approach a difficult discussion, all you may be able to accomplish is to plant a seed. Don't expect to get a positive response right away. Changes are scary, especially to seniors. You may have to wait until they have returned to a more relaxed state to consider your ideas, even if that takes a day or two.

It's also critical to understand that no single response or technique will work to ease tension in every situation. You will need to consider your loved one, the circumstances, and the overall context of the upsetting event. You likely already know some of your family member's triggers and should try to stay away from these when having important or difficult discussions.

If your loved one tends to get overly upset on a regular basis, you may want to study and apply some of the additional techniques recommended by professionals who specialize in de-escalation. You can find many helpful online articles written by nurses, social workers, and psychologists discussing how to de-escalate tense situations with people. The book *De-escalate: How to Calm an Angry Person in 90 Seconds or Less* by Douglas Noll teaches simple techniques that can be used to quickly de-escalate any situation.

Using Positive Self-talk

Realizing that frequent changes are a given for caregivers, we can adjust our self-talk to ease our frustration. Instead of thinking "Oh, no! Now he needs to see the doctor today on top of everything else," we can pivot to "The plan has changed, which is frustrating, but I will make it work." Over time I've begun to be more aware of the thought process I use to get myself through upsetting events or alterations in plans. Here is a process that works for me:

» Take a few deep breaths to calm myself.
» Avoid making quick decisions (except calling 911 during a medical emergency).

» Acknowledge my own frustration or disappointment as well of that of my patient.

» Think through possible options.

» Develop a *new* plan and share it with my patient. If possible, develop the plan *with* my patient.

» Look for silver linings. Is there anything about the change that I can be grateful for?

Helping Patients to Stay Positive

It can be tricky to go through this internal process while also trying to deal with your patient's emotional needs. When upsetting situations occur, I try to keep my demeanor as upbeat and optimistic as possible, and let my patient know we'll figure things out together.

It's important to share your positive energy with your loved one instead of taking on their negative energy. It requires solid self-esteem and confidence, though. If you're feeling good, it's easier to combat the negative energy coming from someone else. Reducing your own stress is key. As you'll read about in Chapter 12, there are many ways to do so, including reading, meditating, and going to therapy.

The following stories show the types of challenges that can arise for caregivers that require them to be flexible:

Singing in the Shower

One beautiful, young, forty-year-old client, Julie, was stricken with early Alzheimer's. At one point her at-home care became too overwhelming and difficult for her family to manage on their own, so she was moved into an assisted living facility. It was designed especially for those with memory loss, so many prompts from staff members helped her manage, and she seemed relatively happy there.

One problem that arose within the first week, however, is that she refused a shower and became combative. The staff tried many ways to help her accept one, but she became belligerent each time. She was incontinent so it was important for her to shower, and she really needed to have her hair washed. She could walk on her own, but she was a fall risk. The family asked if I could intervene in some way. Julie knew me well as I had visited her regularly as a family support when she still lived at home.

The next morning, while she was still in her nightgown, I asked the aide to prepare the shower down the hall with all the items Julie would need. I put her small stereo nearby to play the kind of music she liked best. (She was very fond of music and usually responded positively to it.) I asked the aide to be ready to help me when I brought Julie to the shower.

Julie took my hand and we walked peacefully down the hall and right into the shower room. She became tense until I turned on an upbeat song and started to dance with her. The music distracted her enough that I walked her right into the shower and asked the aide to begin washing her as I removed her nightgown. At first, I thought I could just direct Julie into the shower, but she pulled me in with her—what a surprise! She kept looking at me as we sang and laughed while I washed her hair. Of course, I got soaking wet, but this was an important goal for her, so I set my own comfort aside. Finally, she was clean and wrapped in a warm towel and was very agreeable to getting dressed. We all were amazed that she kept focused on the music enough to stay calm. It all worked out and the aides were so happy to have an idea to try the next time.

The new plan from then on was to recreate that scene with the music on. One aide would dance with her and another help wash her. We soon incorporated plastic gowns for the caregivers to keep them dry during the process. Eventually, Julie seemed to adjust to the idea of an occasional shower.

As a reminder, if this plan had only worked for a minute or two, we would have stopped and tried again later. We knew not to be rigid or physically manipulate her because she would start to cry or become belligerent. This is a solution-oriented story but also one of flexibility, as we needed to open our minds to trying another way. What a relief for all of us that it worked so well!

Oh No, I Sent Her Away!

Once, an aide called me from the hallway of her client's building and said that her client, Eliza, (who had memory loss) had asked the aide to leave the apartment. She told her she was not needed. I asked the aide to stay in the hallway until I called Eliza. Once I got her on the phone, she said, "I want to fire Harriet."

"So, Marie isn't working out for you?" I asked.

"Oh, yeah," she replied, "I meant to say Marie."

This was my way of not drawing attention to the fact that she had used the wrong name. I could have said, "You called her the wrong name," or "You must mean Marie instead of Harriet." When dealing with someone who has memory loss or really anyone who has said the wrong thing, as long as you know what they mean, it doesn't matter what they said. (But verify to be sure that you understood correctly.)

Then I said, "Oh, I thought you were going to the grocery store today." (I did not agree with her that her aide was not needed. Instead, I mentioned the help that Eliza would agree was needed). Eliza agreed that, yes, she had indeed planned to go shopping.

I said, "Usually Marie drives you there and she can hold the umbrella since it's sprinkling out there today."

"Oh no," she said, "I sent her away." I suggested that perhaps she could still catch her in the hallway. Eliza yelled out the front door and Marie returned to the apartment to help.

It was hard for Marie to stay in the apartment when the patient wanted her out, but Eliza needed twenty-four-hour oversight, so it was imperative that someone be with her. She was often sending Marie away, and both she and I had to be flexible so that we could maintain peace yet keep the patient safe. Gradually, over time, Eliza became accustomed to having Marie there, which made everything easier. Initially though, we both knew that we needed to adjust our plans and come up with creative solutions depending on Eliza's feelings on any given day. As a family caregiver you may receive similar phone calls and need to come up with a way to solve the issues peacefully.

Are You Going to Kidnap Me?

One of my patients, Anna, was afraid to leave her home because she thought someone would hurt her. It took some time initially for her to begin to trust me, but slowly, using some of the techniques described in Chapter 6, it began to happen. I found a physician for her and set up an appointment. She still was afraid to go out, so I offered to be with her the whole time and to bring her home if she became uncomfortable. Essentially, I agreed to be flexible depending on her fear level. Finally, she seemed ready and agreed to visit the doctor with my help.

On the day of the appointment, as we approached her door to exit her home, she began to panic. She became red in the face and loudly voiced, "Are you going to kidnap me?" I was quite shocked by her question! I paused briefly to collect myself and somehow managed to calmly respond, "Well, I've never done that before, so I'm not sure I would know how to do something like that."

She calmed immediately and said, "Okay, let's go."

I was amazed that it worked. I remember in that moment thinking about all of the times that I've been scared and wished that someone could have helped me get through it. When we help another person, we help ourselves as well. I was quite concerned that the day would not be successful once her anxiety became elevated but was pleasantly surprised by her trust in me.

Most of us would likely try to *stop* this line of questioning with something like, "No, of course I'm not going to kidnap you!" Instead, we can remove the threat by redirecting the question. I reassured Anna that even if I wanted to kidnap her, I would not know how to do it. This redirection can be more effective than trying to stop someone's thought, especially when there are underlying psychological issues.

By handling it as I did, I acknowledged that it was okay for her to wonder whether I was going to kidnap her. I didn't invalidate her or make her feel worse by suggesting that it was a crazy thought. I also didn't try to stop her from having it. I just wanted to make the day easier for her so we could accomplish the important task of getting her to see a doctor.

Let's Grab Some to Take with Us

On one visit, I took a husband and wife, Harry and Hilda, to a grocery store. As Hilda was picking out bananas, Harry started cracking open peanuts from the display and eating them. Both of them had memory loss, although his was more severe.

I noticed a few shoppers staring at him since he was eating in the store. I remained calm and said, "Let's grab some to take with us." He and I put some peanuts in a bag, including the leftover crumbs. Instead of overreacting, I kept moving forward normally. Redirecting his energy helped the process flow and elicited a non-defensive response. I've learned to expect the unexpected and react calmly, especially with people with memory loss. If you tend to be concerned about what other people will think, this may be hard for you at first. I believe that if others knew the details of the situation, they would understand, so there is no need to be embarrassed or frustrated. Instead, we can simply accept what has happened and move on as best we can.

We're Not Staying at Your Friend's House

Another time, I took a couple, Al and Renee, to a nice beach town an hour away and we had a great day. I had lined up a bed and breakfast for them for an overnight stay. In the evening, I drove them to the B&B, and Renee, who had dementia, said, "Oh, no dear, we're not staying at your friend's house." I tried everything I could to help her understand that a B&B was a different type of lodging, but it just wasn't going to work. Al was fine, but Renee just couldn't grasp the concept. Finally, I had to give in to her concerns and drive them home at ten o'clock that night. As I said, often my techniques work, but you can't win them all. Having a backup option always relieves the pressure of a situation, even if the backup is to give up the current plan and figure out something else entirely. My flexibility allowed me to concede that my plan for an overnight stay had not worked, but I got them home safely and was happy that they had had such a fun day.

She Didn't Notice the Holes

One of my patients, Millie, had once been able to knit beautifully, but her daughter had recently begun noticing holes in some of her work. She thought her mother should give up the activity. My thought was that we should not focus on the holes at all. The accomplishment Millie felt and the good therapy of keeping her hands and fingers moving far outweighed the beauty of the final object. If Millie had noticed the holes herself and felt bad about it, we would have worked together to mend those areas.

People's skills can decline with age, and we have to change our expectations accordingly. When we strive for perfection or expect others to do things exactly as they have in the past, it becomes frustrating and many give up completely. I like to concentrate on the *feeling* of their pursuits and the immediate joy it gives them rather than expecting them to produce a masterpiece. We can learn to be flexible and accepting of mistakes in order to allow our loved ones to do what they are able to do, as long as they are enjoying it.

You're Very Nice, But...

Martha, a home care patient, fell and was hospitalized. Her primary nurse had just gone on vacation for two weeks, so I filled in to help Martha after her fall. Martha was a person who felt more comfortable if everything was done in the *exact* same manner each time. In fact, she demanded it. I was aware of her need for precision and knew some of her habits, but not all of them, so she often had to describe to me exactly how to help her. She said to me, "Of all the times, now when I'm here in the hospital, the person I rely on is on vacation. You're very nice, but you don't know how I need things to be." I really wanted to comfort her but recognized that she was right. I was new and didn't fully understand her desires—she would need to do extra work explaining her needs to me, which increased her anxiety.

I could have said, "Oh, we'll figure it out. I'm capable—it'll be alright" (basically implying that she was worrying too much), but instead

I said, "Oh, I would hate it if that happened to me!" (I didn't tell her she had to *think* differently, but that we'd get through this together.) My response helped her realize that I at least understood her dilemma.

Recognizing—and accepting—what something is like from the other person's point of view is a critical way of demonstrating your respect for them. Patients are allowed to feel and express their frustration, or fear, or any other emotion. In this story, if I didn't want to accept Martha's point of view, it would have likely increased the stress for both of us. But for me, my main concern has always been what the patient needs.

Sometimes we think we are comforting the other person when we're really comforting ourselves. Telling someone not to worry is a great example. It's so important to find out what their needs are and respect them. Though I wasn't her first choice, Martha gradually began to understand that I was on her side and would work hard to be there for her for those two weeks. Recognizing the discomfort she was feeling, I knew I needed to be flexible enough to do things the way she requested in order to ease her anxiety.

───────────

Caregivers are constantly challenged to be flexible, and it can be really hard to accomplish that, especially when stressed. Living with the imbalance of a caregiving relationship takes strength and selflessness. Choosing to be flexible and kind is a courageous act. We must dig deep for the sake of our loved one's health, safety, and comfort. They need us to be willing to provide support when they aren't feeling well or are agitated about a change in plans or circumstances.

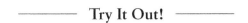

Key Takeaways

» Expect the unexpected! Develop a flexible mindset that allows you to handle changes with grace.

» Often caregivers need to be the ones to adapt—it is too hard for many seniors to change.

» People who are flexible tend to be some of the happiest and most successful in life and at work.

» We are all difficult for someone we interact with because we are all different from one another.

» Use de-escalation techniques to transfer your sense of calm to your loved one so that you can have a more reasonable discussion.

» "Make yourself busy" with other tasks if you need a break from a difficult conversation.

» There is more than one way to accomplish something. Lean toward doing things their way when possible.

» Plans and schedules are helpful but be open to changing them if needed.

» Positive self-talk and optimistic language with your loved one can help smooth difficult situations.

Try It Out!

Think of how you typically react when there is a
sudden change. Look for ways to become more
flexible so that you can adapt more readily.

CHAPTER TEN

BE SOLUTION ORIENTED

In Chapters 8 and 9, I mentioned some behaviors aging adults engage in that require our patience and flexibility. Issues arise daily in senior care, and one of the other major skills caregivers need to develop is the ability to problem solve, often at a moment's notice. Throughout this book, I have emphasized that problem-solving is made substantially easier if your relationship with your family member is characterized by the values we're discussing. Even when you are aware of this, you still need to solve the problems themselves! This chapter explores how to get buy-in for creative solutions that can work for everyone.

Remember that choosing non-defensive wording is part of the solution. Change is difficult for older people, and so as caregivers we have to change ourselves to adapt. When we use calming language, it helps keep everyone relaxed while we're trying to work through problems.

Growing up in a large family with limited resources, I often had to figure things out on my own. My mother would often encourage us to "wing it." My dad would say, "Where there is a will, there is a way." I often helped out with the younger children, and I learned early on how to take care of others, determine what they needed, and help problem solve with them. This background taught me to be resourceful, determined, and persistent, which are probably the attributes that have helped me the most in my role as a care manager.

It is my belief that there is a solution to every problem, but finding one can be daunting. I grew up learning that in any situation, if something isn't working you have to try another way, then another, and then another...until you find a way that does work. According to a quote often attributed to Thomas Edison, "When you have exhausted all possibilities, remember this—you haven't."

One way to be more effective at dealing with problems is to be selective and intentional about prioritizing which problems to tackle. You can't fix every problem. When I worked at my first hospital job, I learned about *triage*, which is the practice of addressing the most serious problem first during first aid care. This concept can be applied to many aspects of caregiving.

Over the years I became adept at thinking of creative ideas on the fly. I was often willing to try unconventional solutions that I'm not sure others would have been comfortable with. You'll read about some of those ideas in the stories included in this chapter. When I look back, I can't remember how I even came up with some of them, but I think it was my belief that there simply *must* be a way to work things out. Don't dismiss your own creative ideas thinking they don't have merit.

I was often surprised when they actually worked! Of course, many of my ideas didn't work out. In this book, for the most part I've only included the ones that did, in the hopes that some of them will work for you too. If the first thing you try isn't successful, don't give up. You will come up with another workable option.

As a nurse, I developed a process for very quickly assessing and naming problems, acknowledging how I felt about them, looking for the cause, and finally coming up with one or more solutions to try. In the following sections, I will walk you through each of these basic problem-solving steps so that you can use this process as well.

Identifying and Naming the Problem

Identifying the problem helps you narrow down which solutions you are going to consider—the solutions for forgetfulness are likely to be different from the solutions for anger. Being able to "name it" will help you focus on ideas that are more likely to work, though many issues can overlap. The following are some of the problems that caregivers often run into with aging loved ones:

- » Resistance
- » Defensiveness
- » Unwillingness to discuss issues
- » Anger
- » Forgetfulness
- » Confusion
- » Unsafe conditions

Acknowledging Your Thoughts and Feelings

When faced with an overwhelming problem, especially resistance, it's natural for caregivers to have these types of feelings and reactions:

- » "I have tried everything."
- » "They are too difficult to work with."
- » "I just need to get away from this situation."
- » "I am really trying, so why won't they try?
- » "I am so frustrated."
- » "They won't listen to good suggestions."
- » "They say no before I even finish a statement."
- » "They say they want to be safe but won't allow any safety measures."

I've had them myself, often. The feelings are completely normal and necessary to recognize. Sometimes we just need a moment to let the feelings surface and admit that we're angry or upset. But once we take time to acknowledge them to ourselves, we need to be able to move beyond them so we can begin to consider some solutions.

Finding the Root Cause

Because we understand how or why *we* do things, it's frustrating when our loved ones won't cooperate with our ideas. It would be so simple if they would just do things our way so we could get them done! But we have to remember that they are adults with their own ideas.

Often the disconnect is that we haven't gotten to the bottom of what is actually happening. We need to fully understand the problem and what is blocking our solutions before a workable plan can be put in place. Sometimes we need to work backward to get to the bottom of an issue. This is when we need to turn to our motivational interviewing again.

After I acknowledge my frustration to myself, my next thoughts about my patient include:

» Will this require them to exert too much energy?
» Does it feel hard for them to try something unfamiliar?
» Will it make them feel unable to be independent or think on their own anymore?
» Is it actual resistance to a new way of doing things, or are they experiencing some anxiety or depression that's holding them back?
» Are they simply overly tired?

These next thoughts are hard to imagine when we're already angry with a person. So often when I've felt this level of frustration, I've had to remind myself that my ultimate goal—to move toward a good outcome—*can* overcome my anger. It truly can. Remember to give yourself a break if you slip up, but then just keep trying.

In order to find a good solution, it helps to find out what is causing the resistance. You can use the tools you learned about in Chapter 2 to figure out your loved one's thought process and work to understand what contributes to their way of thinking.

Much as we go to medical professionals for help, when they ask us to make lifestyle alterations to improve our conditions, we can get prickly. This is true for our family members as well. I have mentioned that none of us like to be told what to do, even if it's for our own good. It seems to bring out our rebellious inner teenager. A University of Michigan white paper on motivational interviewing addresses this "rebellion" phenomenon. The key elements of the researchers' technique for helping to soften peoples' defenses are: 1) emphasizing collaboration, 2) helping someone identify their own reasons for change, and 3) keeping the responsibility for change with them (or in the case of aging loved ones, on you with their input).

Changing your wording so that it reduces potential defensiveness will encourage your family member to talk openly about their needs and what issues feel like to them. Choosing words carefully makes an incredible difference. It will help you better understand what actions on your part will be helpful.

Considering Possible Solutions

Once your understanding is more complete about the underlying cause, you're ready to work on possible solutions. Remember that you don't have to solve everything yourself, although you might be tempted and think it will be the most expedient way.

The best solutions result when you and your loved one consider options together. If you find that they are unable to contribute ideas, start with ones you think they will respond well to. There's always a way to make things work. If you act as a facilitator to solve problems together, you will come up with the answers. Continue to discuss ideas until you both choose a possible solution or until your loved one agrees to try at least one idea.

I mentioned earlier in the book that outside-the-box solutions have often seemed to work the best for me. Somehow, I had a knack for thinking of possibilities other people had not yet thought to try. I believe a large part of this was from my determination to solve the problem. I always had the attitude that it didn't hurt to try something, even if that idea was quite unorthodox, like my dancing and singing in the shower with Julie in the story from Chapter 9. I felt that in the worst-case scenario we would just be back where we started, so why not try?

It can be helpful to use your gut-level, intuitive mind first, to see if there is a solution that feels right. Then follow up with your investigative mind to back up your intuition with facts. I always loved reading Nancy Drew books when I was young. When I'm problem-solving, I often think of myself as a detective trying to solve a case. Here are some helpful techniques I employ as I search for workable answers:

Don't discount short-term solutions. Remember that they are at least an initial step and shouldn't be discounted just because they won't work forever. This may seem counterintuitive. Don't you want to actually solve the entire problem? Yes, but short-term solutions are still solutions. They keep the ball rolling and create momentum. They solve issues now to give you the time and flexibility to work on a better solution or to solve a bigger issue later. Small gains build on themselves and help establish trust. Early small successes help your patient or loved one to see that you are listening, respecting them, and are interested in helping them. Be patient and kind during the process. Sometimes it may take a few days to consider options and come to the best solution.

Limit it to a trial run. Try shrinking the decision by limiting it to something manageable. I often talk with patients about trying something just for a short time to evaluate its effectiveness for them. If it is not helpful or they are not comfortable with it, then we can come up with another idea. I myself like trial runs so that I'm not trapped with any solution that does not work for me. I bet you feel the same way. Similarly, trial runs seem more palatable to most people. They may be willing to try something as long as it can be reversed, which gives them a sense of control. Making decisions that you are going to potentially have to live with forever is always going to be more challenging than deciding to give something a go for a little while.

Avoid strict timelines. In general, as caregivers we want to fix things quickly so that we can be relieved and check them off our list. This is only natural. However, we can actually become more stressed when we try to move too fast to solve problems. I find that more can be accomplished by being patient and flexible. Solutions do not always have to be immediate, even though that might feel better to us. Pushing too hard to hit an artificial timetable adds a lot of stress to an already complicated situation.

Move quickly once there is a consensus. This can help avoid having your loved one change their mind. (Think back to Chapter 2 and the story of Alice, the patient who loudly insisted she couldn't breathe around carpeting. As soon as I secured Alice's permission, I wheeled her straight to her room, which wasn't carpeted.) This method seems to use the energy of their latest agreement to propel them to action. Waiting often causes a setback and a re-evaluation, which can often eliminate a really good idea. Some new ideas are scary so moving forward quickly lessens the time of fearfulness.

These things all involve judgment calls and balance. You can rely on your intuition to tell you when to hold off and when to nudge a little. Often there is no right answer—you know your loved one best, including how they tend to react to change.

Always have another option prepared. Even once we have things figured out and have made a plan, it's good to remember that things can turn south and we might need to pivot to something else. I'm always thinking, "If this doesn't work, then what?" At our staff meetings we'd say, "Okay, that's the plan, and we'll do everything we can to make it work smoothly. But if it doesn't, what is the alternative?" If you think of more than one way to go, you can avoid having your loved one get anxious or stressed out as you try to come up with new ideas on the spot. Sometimes the alternate plan is to just go slower with baby steps if a bigger jump isn't feasible at the moment. Sometimes it's a completely different plan.

Only suggest solutions you know are possible. It's a good idea to get out there and do the legwork first to figure out what can be done. For example, if I'm going to suggest that someone move into an assisted living facility, I want to know where there are slots open. If I'm going to suggest that they hire a driver, I'm going to have some names ready to go. Once you gain buy-in and consensus to do a trial run, you want to be able to make it happen quickly so that the change feels smooth and seamless.

Take a break when you get stuck. When you feel blocked, sometimes the most helpful thing you can do is step away for a moment. Even though you may be desperate for a breakthrough, rather than doggedly continuing to focus on the problem—exhausting yourself in the process—find a quiet place and allow yourself some solitude. Relax and zone out. Focus on your inner thoughts, but not on the problem itself. Or do something unrelated, particularly an activity that lifts your spirits. Try doing something that requires a little bit of physical energy, such as preparing lunch or taking a walk. Maybe listen to some music.

All these strategies relax the conscious mind, which allows the unconscious mind to keep working on the problem to find the solution. You may be thinking "Who has time for that?" But even a few moments away from the situation can help relax your mind, which helps you solve problems, and that, in turn, frees up more of your time. Walking away from the problem for a bit is not a time cost, it is a time investment that will pay dividends.

Trying One Potential Solution at a Time

When families can't agree on a solution, see if they are willing to try one person's action plan first, and if it doesn't work, to try the next person's suggestion. There can only be one idea implemented at a time, so ask the family to support the first choice and evaluate the result. If it is effective, see if they can all agree to continue to support it. Remind everyone that the key is to work together, even if working together means taking turns.

With patience and thoughtful communication, family members can often successfully handle the scenarios I've mentioned in this chapter. If you run into one or more roadblocks and really can't figure out what to do, it may be time to call in a professional. In my experience, there are pronounced differences when a care manager talks with a patient versus a son or daughter trying to discuss the exact same topic with them. Professionals have a bit of healthy distance—they don't have the deep emotional background that comes from growing up with the person. Your loved one may react differently to them even on topics you have tried to talk with them about over and over.

If you are financially able to, consider utilizing a care manager to help with a family member who is uncooperative. They will provide some needed relief for you and can also be a valuable problem-solving resource as you talk through your issues and share ideas. To find one, contact the Aging Life Care Association, a national association that provides assistance with locating a care manager in your area.

The following stories might spark some ideas for creative solutions to use with your loved one:

Who the Hell Are You?

I had the opportunity to meet Evelyn, an incredible woman with memory loss. She lived alone in her house after her husband died. In her life, she had attained three master's degrees—in nutrition, health, and education—and had taught for many years in a one-room schoolhouse. She was just a delightful person, and I grew to really love and enjoy her, especially her Southern accent.

Although Evelyn had a sister, she lived many miles away and was also aging so she could no longer travel. Since no other family lived close by, Evelyn's husband had arranged for a lawyer to manage her affairs. After the husband's death, the lawyer became her friend and visited her often. They thought of each other as family. This was an amazing gift for them both.

One day the lawyer received a call from Evelyn's neighbor, who said that something was wrong. Evelyn was apparently acting strangely and seemed to be losing her memory. He went to visit her right away and found that she seemed perfectly normal. Then another neighbor called and told him the same thing, that Evelyn was acting as though she didn't know where she was. He went again and found her to be normal. But on another day when he visited, he found that she didn't know him and wanted to know what he wanted. What a shock! How was this possible?

He stayed with her and placed a call to me to ask for help in her care. Fortunately, I was available to go over right away, but on my arrival, she recognized the lawyer again. She was quite cordial to me—she introduced me to her lawyer friend while he sat puzzled. I told Evelyn about my role as a care manager and explained that I would help her whenever the lawyer was not available. She understood and agreed but explained that although she was pleased to meet me, she was doubtful she would ever need me.

The next day I surprised her with a visit, and as she opened the door, she said, "Who the hell are you?" I explained that her lawyer had sent me, and she replied, "I don't have a lawyer." I let her know that he had asked me to find out if she had all the medications she needed. "What?" she asked, "Of course I do."

I asked her to allow me to see the medications just in case. To my amazement, she let me in and showed me where she kept them. We started to chat, and she told me stories about her husband and showed me his picture. I noticed that she had her lunch (a sandwich) on the table, so I told her that I was going to leave but would return another time.

I called the lawyer to explain that although her memory seemed to fluctuate, she seemed able to dress herself and prepare her lunch safely. We talked about getting twenty-four-hour care for her if she would accept it. It was a long process, and it took many days of encouraging her to have someone with her. Her lawyer told her that he wanted someone there at least during winter to shovel the walk and take out the trash since it was no longer safe for her. She trusted him so much and loved his visits, so she complied.

I arranged for her to see a neurologist, and he was baffled in the beginning. He checked to see if seizures were causing the changes in her, but after testing he found no evidence of that. After many other tests, he determined that she had Lewy body dementia, which can initially cause fluctuating memory and cognition. Sometimes she was normal for days and then abruptly changed to not knowing much at all.

My role was to help Evelyn's aides understand her condition and to consider ideas to keep her safe and healthy. I also took her to her oncologist for regular appointments (she was a cancer survivor). The oncologist agreed to become her primary physician so that she would have fewer changes in physicians.

One day, I took her to the oncologist, and she seemed quite normal and told him how much she loved him. She thanked him for helping her heal from cancer. On the way home from that appointment, she said she was getting a headache. Then, suddenly, she didn't know where she was anymore. I told her I was driving her to her home and that she would be more comfortable there.

When we arrived at her home, she refused to get out of the car. She said, "It's the wrong house," and started to become agitated. Rather than insisting it was her house and trying to take her in, I thought of a way to try to avoid a confrontation entirely.

First, I said, "Well, let me check just in case." Then, I got out of the car, locked it, and went into her home (the lawyer had given me a key). I made her the same sandwich she always made for lunch and put half of it on the same type of plate she always used.

I took the sandwich to the car—favorite plate and all—and showed it to her. "This looks like your sandwich. It was on the table," I told her. She took a bite of it and said, "Yes, this is mine." While I hoped the sandwich and plate would be familiar to her and relax her, I was also thinking that she might be hungry and would perhaps think more clearly if she ate something. Fortunately, she wanted to eat the sandwich as soon as she recognized the plate.

Afterward, I encouraged her by saying, "Let's go inside and check it out." She agreed to enter the home with me. I was initially quite concerned that it would be a struggle to get her out of the car, and as I have said, my philosophy is never to force people. Even though she was very petite, she was quite strong. What a relief for us both that she agreed to come with me. Feeding her had allowed me to redirect her back into the house where there was another half sandwich waiting for her. She still seemed a bit uncertain once inside but remained calm.

The aides and I worked very hard to think of ways to help her life stay peaceful when she didn't understand her situation on her poor memory days. We started very slowly with aides visiting just a few hours a day and gradually increased her care until the full twenty-four hours were covered. It would have been wonderful to have started twenty-four-hour care immediately, but I suspected that Evelyn would respond better to a slow adjustment. Sometimes implementing something right away works, but in this situation, we needed to be flexible. The lawyer and I stayed in close contact with her during the transition to make sure she remained safe.

I knew that the journey for Evelyn to accept twenty-four-hour care would take some time. She began to trust me early on and allowed me to assist her with laundry and other chores. After a few days, I told her I was not available but would send my friend (an aide). Once she adapted to that aide, she became accepting of having another aide at night. Slowly, but surely, she accepted the safety of round-the-clock care at home. When she was clear headed, she requested that she remain in her home for as long as possible. The lawyer and I both supported that choice, and she was able to stay at home until she passed in her own bed many years later.

As this story demonstrates, some patients' situations are very complex, requiring problem-solving on many levels. There is so much to learn about memory loss, which is why many caregiving books are dedicated to the topic. On the day I took Evelyn to see the doctor, I was so glad I remembered that showing a person with memory loss something they recognize can sometimes bring them back to the present long enough to be calmed.

May I Use Your Bathroom?

I loved being with a beautiful young client of mine, Rose, who had early-onset Alzheimer's disease. She was so gentle and smiled almost all of the time. Before her illness, she had trained animals to be care companions, so she had a warm heart for animals as well as people.

Her husband, Peter, took a leave of absence to be with her more as her memory deteriorated. They both did well together due to their long relationship and his extreme patience. After some time though, he began to need more help and found that it was difficult for others to care for her, as she did not always respond to their guidance.

He called me because he took Rose for a walk every day and it was becoming more difficult to get her to turn around when it was time to return home. She started resisting more and more, as she wanted to keep walking. He seemed to manage a way each time but was hopeful that a caregiver could begin helping out. He was not having success finding someone who was able to take her for a walk and then help her turn around and head back home. They had to call him for help every time.

I asked for Peter's permission to take Rose out so that I could see her behavior when it was time to go home. We walked a long way and then it was time to turn around. I motioned for us to start back, but she began to pull me to continue on. I then whispered in her ear, "May I please use your bathroom?" She looked at me compassionately and immediately turned back to her house. I was shocked, but it proved that she still maintained her ability to be socially accommodating for a guest. It might not be possible to use that method every single day, but it showed that there was at least one peaceful way to accomplish the task. I resolved to think of even more options after my initial success.

Rose continued to live at home with her husband until her care became more complicated and it became obvious that a memory care center was a more appropriate place for her to reside. At the center we found for her, there was a central enclosed area where she could walk and walk and never have to turn around to go home—she loved that. She even seemed to relate to some of the other people there. Her husband and I both continued to visit often to make sure she was comfortable.

This was another scenario where I was glad I remembered that tapping into some aspect of prior behavior (like good manners, entrenched over a lifetime) can sometimes help when working with people with memory loss.

Trade With Me

A patient named Maude who had memory loss loved to go out to eat with her husband, Nick. He had memory loss as well. Neither of them was allowed to drive anymore so I would take them out, and it was fun for us. She was a very elegant lady and enjoyed dressing up for the occasion. She was clearly able to read the menu and choose her dinner and would even ask questions of the waiter.

When the meal was served, however, her memory loss kicked in and she would tell the waiter: "This dinner is not what I ordered." He would calmly reply that her meal was what he wrote down as her request. She would say, "No it isn't," and start to become agitated. I knew from previous experience what entrees she liked, so I always ordered one of those for myself. When she complained about her meal, I would say, "Here, Maude, trade with me." She would agree, taste a few bites, and then say, "Now this is what I should have ordered."

This occurred on a regular basis. Nick would say, "Maude, just eat it." She told him that she wanted what she ordered. To help her enjoy the evening without an upset, I routinely made the trade. It did not seem to bother her, even though it happened time and time again, because she quickly forgot about each exchange.

I didn't mind the trade, and it allowed them to have an enjoyable meal with minimal conflict. So often when you are caring for someone with memory loss, if you are flexible, you will be able to think of solutions that will allow your loved one to stay calm and even enjoy themselves.

You'll Take Me Out?

Another patient on our memory loss unit at the nursing home, George, needed blood work. When the lab technician came to draw his blood, he became agitated and refused to cooperate. George didn't know the lab technician and did not seem to understand what was about to happen. They were very patient with him, but after a few days of getting the same reaction over and over, I saw the need for a new approach. I took an aide with me and brought all the blood work supplies when I went to his room.

I sat next to him and said, "I keep seeing you at the door and it seems like you want to go out for a walk." He nodded. I told him I would take him out for a walk as soon as he had his blood drawn. I let him know the doctor needed to have the results to know if his medication was at the right level. He said, "You'll take me out?" and I responded, "I sure will! Right after we finish this."

He knew me, which helped. When I held his arm in position for a blood draw, he actually held still and allowed me to perform the task. I then handed the tray of vials and supplies to the aide to take to the other nurse, and I walked with him outside of the locked unit right away. It was a nice sunny day. I was concerned that he might not return with me, but fortunately when I told him that lunch was being served, he turned around and went back inside with me. I was thrilled since I really did not know what to expect—he was a very tall, strong man and I'm not sure I could have forced him back even if I'd wanted to—but it all worked out beautifully. I could have called for help if I needed it, but I was trying to keep things as comfortable for him as possible. Too many people trying to get him to return would likely have been a traumatic experience for him, and he may have formed negative associations with me or with getting his blood drawn, either of which would have made things more difficult later on.

Often the solution to reluctance on the part of a patient is to consider an incentive for them. In this case, George accepted the procedure in order to be able to go for the walk he wanted.

I Won't Fall

A favorite uncle of mine was ready for discharge from a rehab center to his home. Prior to rehab, he was hospitalized after a fall. He was anxious to go home and be with my aunt—they loved each other very much.

My uncle's family said they would arrange twenty-four-hour care at home since he could not yet walk and was confined to a bed or chair. He absolutely refused to agree to care at home and became angry with his family for pushing the idea. He felt that my aunt would not like having someone else in the home.

His family asked for my input. I thought he was likely just trying to protect my aunt. In reality, though, she had agreed to be his caregiver to keep him happy without realizing everything caregiving would involve. I have often seen this, especially when couples care so much and want to be there for each other. My uncle needed to recognize that my aunt could actually be injured while attempting to help him transfer from one spot to another. He would not like the guilt of her being injured while helping him. It was important to help him realize that the real gift to my aunt would be to relieve her of caregiving duties rather than trying to avoid the bother of having other people in the house. Or at least not to burden her with all the caregiving immediately upon his return so that there would be time to better assess the reality of the situation and determine which duties she might want to take on herself.

His family was focused on the fact that he might fall, but he just said, "I won't," and ended the conversation. Focusing on the possibility of an injury to my aunt, however, made him think more carefully. Often, one partner will make a choice they don't like because they think they are giving their partner what he or she wants. By showing him the possibility that he might be hurting his loved one instead of helping her, I was able to use his own internal motivation (to protect and care for his wife) to lean him toward making a different decision.

Couples are very often willing to do something if it helps their partner. When I'm working toward this, I talk to each of them individually to find out their true feelings about how they think a situation should be handled. Their love for each other often leads them to a good outcome.

That's Exactly What We Need

A physicist named John and his wife, Sandra, had just moved in to a nice, small apartment. Sandra thought she had found a perfect place for them and it even had a little balcony. But then their daughter, who had emotional issues, came with her two dogs and decided to stay to help them out. It felt crowded, and they were uncomfortable with her there but didn't know what to do.

Shortly afterward, John got a urinary tract infection, and had to be hospitalized because he needed IV antibiotics. When he was starting to recover, he was told he'd have to have physical therapy to regain his strength before he could go back home. Often people in his situation are sent to a long-term care facility, but he wanted to be with Sandra. And yet it was so hectic at home. The couple was referred to me by an aide agency over concerns about their situation.

Rather than push him to go to a facility, I got the idea to try to inspire the couple instead. I said, "Wow, you both have so much going on right now. I wish you could go on a vacation."

Sandra said, "Oh, that would be wonderful. Too bad it can't be Hawaii. We'll just have to figure something out."

At that point I suggested they consider going to a facility together. Before I suggested this, I had called around and was lucky to have found one that had a place available in a few days. I told the couple, "Since John needs to have therapy, if you take a vacation to the assisted living facility right next to the hospital, you can be there together and he can get his physical therapy in the same building."

Sandra perked up and said, "Yes, that's exactly what we need." I was able to secure a beautifully furnished place with a monthly rental option and got his doctor's consent. They were accepted and were so pleased when they saw the apartment.

Once they settled in, they wound up really liking it! An aide came and took John to rehab when it was time. The facility had prepared food ready for them at every meal. After a few weeks, I overheard them discussing what to do after he was rehabilitated. I showed them a larger, unfurnished apartment in the same place, and to my surprise, they wound up deciding to move there permanently. The daughter stayed back at the original apartment with the two dogs but was close enough to check on them often.

It was so beautiful to see John and Sandra be open-minded about the idea of taking a vacation to ease their stress. It did turn out to be the perfect time because he needed rehab, and the situation with their daughter likely made them more open to the idea. Since then, I have used the "vacation" idea with other patients, and it has helped at least open them up to other possibilities for their living situation.

―――――――

Even though seniors can be interesting and wise and fun, they also can be a source of tremendous frustration for family members and caregivers. They often refuse safety and health measures even though they are for their own good. They tend to see our advice as interference rather than suggestions made out of love and our desire to protect them. Remembering our goals and using the problem-solving process outlined in this chapter can help reduce the friction and lead to greater cooperation and satisfaction for all.

―――――― **Key Takeaways** ――――――

- » Believe there is a solution to every problem, even if finding it seems daunting.
- » Work to fully understand the problem and what is getting in the way of an effective solution.
- » It helps to identify and name the problem, acknowledge your thoughts and feelings about it, and work to understand the root cause before considering possible solutions.
- » Consider short-term solutions and trial runs as initial steps. Remember that short-term solutions are still solutions!
- » If possible, move quickly once there is a consensus about what to do. It helps to research solutions in advance so that you are ready to spring into action once there is agreement.
- » If you're stuck on a problem, take a short break to relax your mind.
- » Try to think of creative solutions that will elicit calm responses.

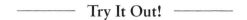

Try It Out!

Think of a current issue you are dealing with in your caregiving role and apply my problem-solving approach to it. Can you identify what is causing the resistance and find a way to address it in order to gain your loved one's cooperation?

CHAPTER ELEVEN
———————

ENJOY THE MOMENT

I've acknowledged throughout this book that caregiving can be difficult, but it can also be wonderful and rewarding! One of the ways we can make caregiving less stressful is by making it a point to enjoy special moments together with our loved one. Sometimes this happens organically during our visits with them, but we can also *create* moments of joy for them. Doing so benefits them, of course, but also helps *us* by making our role more fun.

But how do we help *create* those moments of joy? One simple way is to sincerely be there for them and have their best interest in mind. In Chapter 4, I talked about how important acceptance is in improving their frame of mind. Imagine how wonderful it is for your family member to know that you accept their thoughts and feelings and love them just as they are. That type of connection can be magical and gives everyone a good feeling.

It is easy to miss opportunities for pleasure when we are busy and distracted. Taking some time to appreciate the beauty of flowers, the feeling of fresh air, the change of decor for the season, and other simple moments is worth the effort. We can train ourselves to search for the opportunities for bliss that appear before us each day, especially those that exist in nature. It could be a rainbow after a storm, a beautiful sunset, or the sliver of a recent moon. Noticing and sharing that bliss with your relative is a loving thing to do. For a deeper understanding of how to notice and capitalize on these opportunities, I highly recommend Chip and Dan Heath's book *The Power of Moments: Why Certain Experiences Have Extraordinary Impact*.

Science shows that the practice of paying attention to the good things in our lives, even briefly, can actually make us feel happier months later! We do have to make a point of noticing the joy that we feel, as we are often focused on problems and difficulties instead of more positive emotions. Like the process of acquiring any new skill, we have to make a conscious effort to do it.

Petting an animal, listening to music, or watching an inspiring movie can bring much comfort. Most senior centers offer a variety of entertaining activities. Timing can be important because your loved one may not currently be in the mood to think of positive or beautiful things if they are feeling irritable. At certain times, being reminded of happy things in their life may even feel like they are being pressured to feel better. We can find the right time though. Anything that distracts them from their difficulties, even for a few moments, has the potential to make a difference.

Paying attention and offering these moments of pleasure to the people we care for will improve their lives. If you can redirect them toward fun activities when they are ready, they may be less cranky or less concerned with their current ailments. If your family member is not up for activities at the moment, simply brightening up their surroundings can have just as much of a positive effect on them as it would for us.

We can help people with memory loss experience moments of joy as well. *Creating Moments of Joy Along the Alzheimer's Journey* by Jolene Brackey—a book I highly recommend reading—offers many ideas for providing enjoyment.

Remember that each moment for someone with impaired memory is a new moment.

We can focus our energy on creating more joy for them. One way to do that is to trigger meaningful memories for them. It's fun for all of us to reminisce! Long-term memory stays with people the longest, which gives them an opportunity to relive some happy moments in their mind when we bring them up. Music they loved during their childhood seems to be especially good at bringing out positive emotions.

Recreational therapists are licensed or credentialed health professionals who sometimes work with older people privately in their own homes. It may be worthwhile to invest in a few sessions with one of them for your loved one. Their doctor may be able to refer you to a local therapist. Medicare covers recreational therapy for certain conditions. This type of therapy is an important tool that helps seniors to reconnect with the activities they once enjoyed—or find new ones—in a way that improves their physical and mental health, as well as their cognitive function. The therapists often have many good ideas for drawing out the fun side of patients.

One tip for brightening up the lives of patients or loved ones is to offer them opportunities that they feel are lost to them. I like to offer them what I call "a bigger world" to enjoy, especially by providing opportunities to try something they really wish they could do. Even if it is complex and you think you can only do it one time, granting them their wish once is far better than never doing it at all.

Offering a Bigger World

One way to offer a bigger world is to encourage patients to get outside! So many older people spend their lives living in their apartments or houses and only go out for doctor appointments. Many folks get stuck and think that their lives can no longer be joyful. It makes me so sad. You can help motivate a change in that pattern of thought.

I hear patients say, "I use a wheelchair, and we don't have a ramp, so I can't go out." There are tools such as portable ramps that might be a solution for someone who does not want a permanent ramp. They may imagine that it's too much trouble, but in the end, they will love the feeling of getting outside again. I've seen the look on someone's face after they have been in a hospital and then rehab and then are finally wheeled out into the fresh air. It's so uplifting—a momentary delight!

Seeing the outside world can really elevate one's mood. I am sure you have noticed that feeling after you have been homebound for a few days with the flu and are finally able to be outside again.

Find the reasons your family member thinks they can't do something and consider how valid they are. In Chapter 7, I told the story of Brian, who was confined to his bed and thought to be unlikely to walk again. I related how important it was to help him into a chair for some time every day, especially a chair in another room for some variety. A change of scenery can be very uplifting.

Some might say, "What's the point? A lounge chair is just like the bed." This overlooks the different light and color and space that can be experienced just by being in a different spot in the room or in another room. Over time, some of my patients were able to sit in a chair for longer and longer periods of time and it improved their mood greatly. Unless there is a specific, special circumstance that actually prevents someone from getting up, you might as well try. Looking out from the same bed over and over is so different from sitting in another room with sunshine on your face.

When I listen to patients say what they wish for but cannot have, I think hard about any possible way to fulfill their wish, even if it's just once. For those who truly can't go outside, consider playing video clips on your phone or laptop for them. There are so many fun and amazing videos available on YouTube and other video-sharing sites that show nature, music, meditation, humor, and more. You can offer your family member a bigger world just by letting them see short clips of what's out there.

Providing Special Moments At Least Once

It's okay to have something happen just once! So many caregivers seem to shy away from doing something extra special for patients one time, because they don't want them to "get used to it." Sure, they might want it again, but why not give them that treat now, and maybe even again if at all possible? Just explain in advance that this event is an occasional treat.

That's fine! People go on vacations all the time, which are an occasional treat. You can't discount how amazing that experience might be for someone, especially if you're giving them something they thought they had lost forever.

Small activities that seem to bring great joy to older people include music, massage, art or art therapy, reminiscing, receiving greeting cards, beautiful mild scents, fairy tree lights, and movement such as dance or water therapy. Helping to create moments of joy for your loved one will bring them good feelings, a better mood, and a more cooperative spirit. Even a momentary delight may distract them from any discomforts they may be feeling. If they never get to do an activity again, they may still enjoy reminiscing about their past fun experiences, which is a joy in itself.

Drawing Out Their Interests

You will notice when you read the stories in this chapter that I do not tell my patients which activities to try. Saying, "Why don't you try music, or knitting, or getting in touch with your friends," can feel to them that they are not doing what they should be doing in life. Often families use those directive words to try to be helpful, and I appreciate how well meaning they are. For some people though, directive words can seem like extra pressure. What I try to do is find their voice within and bring it out. I always say, "I wonder what it would be like if this happened?" Again, they don't have to answer at all if they don't want to. It gives them unpressured time to think about it.

Here are a few stories about ways you can bring more joy into someone's life:

A Slice of Heaven

Edna, who was 96 years old and lived in an independent living residence, told me how much she missed soaking in a warm bath. She had not been able to get in or out by herself for a few years. It had become too difficult for her due to her arthritis. I felt confident that we could do it safely together and suggested we try. At first, she had doubts about my ability to get her back out of the tub, but I could tell she was tempted. She had strong grab bars and surprisingly strong arms, so I really believed we could do it. With good positioning and with my assistance, she was able to experience a comforting bath again.

She couldn't believe it. She said, "I feel like I've just gone to heaven!" It might not have been safe for an untrained person to help her, but nurses and aides are trained in how to maneuver patients safely. Being able to give her that special treat made my day as well.

It's easy to assume that some things are no longer possible once people hit a certain age. But my belief is that the effort is worth it, even if it's just every once in a while. Edna took regular showers with a shower chair, but her real wish was to have the experience of soaking her whole body in water. If I had not been strong enough, I would have arranged for extra help so she could have that "slice of heaven" again.

I Don't Want to Go Alone

My patient, Ida, missed her husband so much. He recently passed away and she was still adjusting to the loss. I visited her to have her sign some papers, and found her crying.

She had just received an invitation to the weekend reunion that she and her husband had attended in previous years. They were part of a group of very close friends that had an annual gathering at a beach house that one of the couples owned. She said, "I'm so sad. I can never go there again since David is gone." I wondered out loud if she would consider going if she had transportation for the two-hour trip. She said, "I don't want to go alone, and I won't go with someone I don't know." Obviously, she wanted to go be with her friends, and I was sure they would be a comfort to her.

She was fortunate that her husband left her with adequate finances to pay privately for assistance. I explained that her care manager, my colleague Catherine, might be able to take her and stay with her. She looked up excitedly and said, "Would she do that? I love being with her."

I placed a call to Catherine and found that she was open and available on the designated weekend. Ida started crying again, but this time with joy. She was just elated! I knew she had a journey ahead in the next few months and years to learn what was possible for her now, but this was a beginning. I was thrilled to be able to offer it to her.

She went to the reunion and was grateful that her friends offered her so much support and warmth. They all vowed to keep in close touch with her. She missed her husband dearly, but she had taken an important first step toward recovery from her loss. She and Catherine bonded even more during that trip, which helped Ida feel less alone.

Although she had no local relatives, if her budget had not allowed for a care manager, I feel sure we could have found her a friend or someone she would at least be comfortable with to accompany her to the reunion. Sometimes we limit our own options unnecessarily as Ida did here, especially when we are emotionally upset or sad. Caregivers can often help a patient think through new and different possibilities.

Can I Play?

Emma, who lived alone in her own home, had become less stable when walking. She was a little lonely and seemed reluctant to go out. She was quite healthy and intelligent but not as agile as she had been in the past, which I'm sure made her feel vulnerable. She resisted stepping out into the world, preferring instead to stay home and avoid new situations and terrain.

Her son Walter was concerned because he thought she would be happier if she had something to do that interested her. He had been unsuccessful thus far in convincing her to try any activities, so he asked me to see if I could help. He was hoping I could brighten her life in some way.

I began visiting her so that she would get to know me and could call me if her son were unavailable. After a few visits, when she became more comfortable, I said to her, "I'm looking for something that's really fun for you to do in this house. What was fun for you when you were a little girl?" She responded, "I know what that is! My mother hated it, but my brother and I played ping-pong on the dining room table." She continued on for some time about how much fun the game was to play.

At my next visit, I told her that I found a place around the corner where we could go watch people play ping-pong. There was no anticipation on my part that she'd do anything more than just watch. With less hesitancy than I expected, she agreed to accompany me to the senior center. Is it possible she always said no when her son asked about activities because she thought she would be inconveniencing him? Had she felt pressured because he was being too directive with his requests? It may simply have been that she just really liked ping-pong and was excited to see it again. Her reasons were unclear to me, but she agreed quickly so we left to check it out.

We drove to the center and began watching some people play. She was so excited! I guess it reminded her of the fun she'd had with her brother. When the room emptied out at lunchtime, she surprised me by asking, "Can I play?" Her voice was full of anticipation. She and I played together, and it was amazing to see how much she enjoyed it. I took a picture of her serving the ball to me and sent it to her son to show him that she was out and playing ping-pong again. He was, of course, totally elated for her.

When Emma had told me about her childhood experience, I watched her eyes light up. I could just *feel* how that memory perked her up. Initially, I thought maybe she and I could play ping-pong on her dining room table to recreate her cherished childhood memory. However, once I remembered that the senior center had ping-pong, it seemed like a good option. It worked out great and we both loved it.

Some type of fun is available at any age. We just have to help our loved ones identify some potential sources of joy on any given day.

Really Having Fun

Even those with memory loss can laugh about certain circumstances, and what a joy that is. On one of my memory loss units in a nursing home, there were two women, Grace and Maria, who seemed to be great friends. They would sit on the couch and mumble incoherent words to one another all day and then just laugh and laugh. I was so touched by their ability to enjoy those moments. It helped me realize that what we may view as sad may actually be joyful to someone with memory loss. We have no way of knowing what their life feels like to them, but the women's laughter gave me the sense that they were really having fun.

Watch your family member for expressions of happiness, contentment, or excitement and notice what tends to trigger them. This will help you know them better and understand what they are feeling, and it will provide you with ideas to help them feel joy more often.

Let's Watch

I took one of my patients, Norma, to the mall to see if that would appeal to her. She liked walking around with me and having lunch, but as soon as she saw the escalator she said, "Let's watch." We found a bench nearby and began looking at the people descending from the escalator.

She seemed to love to make a comment about each of them. "Look at the hat she is wearing. It's so bright!" "Oh, she looks like she better hold on." "Why is he taking two steps at a time? He doesn't have to do that on an escalator." "Oh, that outfit is not appropriate for a mall."

I think she could have stayed there all day focusing on all the things she noticed. What a joy to watch her. Some of her statements were so comical, they could have made a great skit on late night television. Humor is so good for the soul!

Later I asked an aide to take her there occasionally because it was so much fun for her. They watched the people on the escalator for a few moments but then the aide tried to redirect her to looking at the stores. Norma would have none of that! She was having too much fun. Later the aide told me she was frustrated that Norma only wanted to sit and watch when there were a lot more exciting things going on at the mall. I reminded her that the joy Norma felt watching the people come down the escalator is immensely important to her life right now. It lifts her spirits and makes her laugh and helps her to express herself.

Part of our role is to lead our patients toward that joy as much as possible. Even if you don't think what they are enjoying is very fun yourself, you can at least take pleasure in how much you are brightening their life in that moment. Sometimes we need to be patient and be present while our loved one enjoys something. It's important to give them that gift of time.

Maintaining the Feeling

One patient, who was in her late nineties, Bertha, used to do artwork, but thought she was no longer able to do so. She mentioned how frustrated she felt to be less able to paint the way she used to. Some of the beautifully detailed paintings she had done in the past were displayed on her walls. They were absolutely amazing, and for a moment it was sad to think that she was no longer capable of producing that quality.

She and I both agreed that she wanted to maintain that feeling of working with color and creating as she once had. So, on one visit, I brought two painting tablets and some watercolor pens. We decided to paint side by side, making any designs we chose, experimenting with the use of color. She loved it and her spirits lifted immensely.

Eventually I brought her blank note cards that she could paint designs on, and I helped her address the accompanying envelopes and send them to her friends.

Accepting that a small, unique design was beautiful rather than feeling pressured to put detail into a full-size painting eased Bertha's mind. Her use of color was extraordinary and I admired her work so much. The process of being creative led her to feel such joy. Eventually she used many different types of paint pens. The brush pens gave her more control than a brush she had to dip into paint.

Remember that success is a great motivator. It gives seniors a sense of pride in their accomplishments, which will make them want to try to be more autonomous in other areas of their lives.

––––––––––

Instead of focusing on the sadness of a situation like aging, if we open our eyes to the positive aspects of life, there are always many to notice! Often those positives are quite enjoyable. By keeping things light, caregivers can help their patients experience more fun despite their maladies or disabilities. Even just offering a warm smile can be comforting.

As family caregivers, one of the ways we can find joy in our *own* lives is by watching our loved ones enjoy themselves. Just taking a moment here and there to help them appreciate something beautiful can change their point of view and lift their mood, which in turn can have an uplifting effect on us. Try to direct your family member's attention to anything that can potentially bring them joy in the moment.

——— **Key Takeaways** ———

» Try to create moments of joy for your loved one often. It helps them and helps you by making your role more fun.

» Find opportunities to help your family member pet an animal, listen to music, or watch an inspiring movie to bring them comfort and joy.

» Train yourself to search for the opportunities for bliss that appear before you each day, however small, to share with your loved one.

» Show them a bigger world! Offer them a desired activity, even if it can only be done once, to let them feel that moment of joy.

» Take your loved one to reunions and weddings, or play games like ping-pong with them, to add excitement and energy to their life. It may take some planning but can often be accomplished.

» Watch for their expressions of joy as clues to activities that will help them feel that joy more often.

» Help them to experience joy by showing them how to do old activities in new ways.

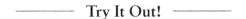

——— **Try It Out!** ———

What is something that your loved one would
really enjoy doing but has given up? Think of
a way to offer it to them again, even if it is a
simpler version or can only be done once.

CHAPTER TWELVE

TAKE CARE OF YOURSELF, TOO

My focus in previous chapters has been primarily on easing and enhancing the interactions you have with your loved one to best ensure their safety and to increase their overall well-being and happiness. In this final chapter, it's time to focus on *you*!

The caregiving journey is often a long one, and the needs of our patients or loved ones typically increase over time. Conscientious caregivers can end up taking their roles so seriously that they can start to lose sight of their own needs. This can happen gradually because it's easy to neglect yourself when you have other major demands on your time. You just go and go until at some point you realize that you are starting to get depleted—or worse, that you are already totally drained. Your empathy for your family member starts fading, and you begin to lose your ability to give to others.

If you've been caring for a loved one for a long time, or you're doing it because there's no one else available, you may be at risk of developing what is called *emotional burnout*. You may find that despite your good intentions, you can no longer just push through. You may feel as though you are in a mental fog.

Sometimes we're slow to realize just how depleted we are. It can happen to even the most resilient of us. Often, it's a result of poor self-talk. We tell ourselves "If I take a break, I'll never get everything done." Or that "Everyone is counting on me and I can't let them down."

I can't stress enough how important it is for you to find some way to refuel and recharge. And don't forget to take care of your own physical health. Getting enough sleep, eating healthy foods, getting periodic exercise, and sharing your struggles with others can all help prevent burnout.

Chronic stress can adversely affect your physical and emotional health as well as the health of your relationships. You don't want to get to the point where you feel compelled to release your tension by yelling at your family member or saying something you'll regret.

There are many ways to take care of yourself along the caregiving journey so you don't reach this point. If you're a reluctant caregiver, you may have an even heavier burden and will need to work a little harder on getting help and practicing good self-care.

There are numerous sources of support available for people who are looking after family members. I will share some of them in this chapter. First let's look at some of the more stressful aspects of caregiving. The first is the tendency of caring people to take on the suffering of their loved one and feel their emotional pain as if it were their own. Also, it's common for caregivers to feel unappreciated by their loved one and other family members. Dealing with criticism from others about how you are giving care makes things worse, especially if those family members aren't actually helping to provide care. Having to take care of a relative when you really don't want to can also bring up a lot of uncomfortable feelings. Emotional support can make all the difference in these circumstances.

Safeguarding Your Energy

As important as it is to show care and concern for others, as caregivers we must also be careful not to "take on" the suffering or pain of our loved ones. Many naturally empathetic and caring people will suffer on behalf of a loved one. This only serves to compound the total suffering, drain our energy, and reduce our ability to provide comfort and ease to the patient. By taking on some of their burdens, we increase them, as now we are both burdened. Caregiving can last months or years, and it's important to take steps to keep up our own stamina and protect our own mental health. We need to find the courage to be able to sit with and witness our family member's pain without "inhabiting it" ourselves so much that we become just another person who is suffering and needs assistance. Life is full of sorrows, and we will all have our turn, but taking on someone else's suffering is both unnecessary and harmful to us. We must continually work on increasing our resilience if we're to handle whatever life throws at us.

Feeling Unappreciated

Family caregivers often don't feel appreciated, which adds to their emotional burden. It's understandable that you'd want some recognition for your efforts, but unfortunately it may not be forthcoming, which can be a source of disappointment and resentment. Someone who is tired, sick, or in pain will be self-focusing and may be unable to let you know how much you are appreciated, even if they are aware of your hard work and commitment to them. You may be looking for some positive feedback from them to help you feel better, but friends or caregiver support groups may have to fill that void until your loved one feels better.

Dealing With Criticism from Family Members

Sometimes our siblings or other relatives, especially out-of-towners, become critical of our care because they don't have the same exposure to the day-to-day issues that we are dealing with. Relatives might also not appreciate all that we do. I have heard so many siblings say they had no idea how big the job was, and that they only felt enlightened when they themselves became more involved and learned how much there was to manage.

Constant suggestions, criticisms, or directives from family and friends can compound the problem for caregivers, even if they are intended to be helpful. Directly involving these individuals can enable them to be more realistic about what is possible. Though everyone is doing their best, family members can be more helpful by pitching in instead of criticizing, but sometimes they need to be invited to do so.

In my own family, as my mom started to need more care but refused a professional caregiver, my sister stepped up to the plate and began managing her needs. It wasn't until my sister—who was also going through multiple other life stresses at the time—started to become anxious, angry, and resentful that we realized that we could all be doing more. We only realized what a burden it had become when my sister was brave enough to ask for help. In response, one of us took over Mom's finances while another one began more medical management. Each of us took one designated night to call Mom on the phone so there wouldn't be too many calls at once. We all started visiting more frequently from out of town. Mom had been missing her children, and our increased attention to her made her feel very happy and loved.

Remember that most people are well meaning and that all members of the family are likely doing their best to help, even when that help seems to come in the form of criticizing what we're doing. While focusing on the person we're caring for, we often forget to think of what we need and what our other family members need. It's important to keep those lines of communication open so that everyone's needs are met and the load can be shared. "Many hands make light work," as they say.

Asking for Help

Feeling alone in your role can be really overwhelming. It will eventually catch up with you by causing you to feel angry or tired or resentful of others you think should be helping but aren't. You may feel that you are responsible because you live the closest to your loved one. I have seen this dynamic play out in many families. Often the primary caregiver feels they have no choice since they are nearby, and other family members are afraid to step in because they think the designated family member wants the responsibility and control. If you are the primary caregiver, you may feel conflicted. You may not want to deal with others' ideas and suggestions, yet it's just too tiring to keep going it alone.

Primary caregivers often feel that others should be *offering* to help, since they feel like they are drowning in their duties. Many people have expressed that sentiment to me. The truth, more often than not, is that *you have to ask for help* when you need it. Whether you actively want to be the primary caregiver or feel you have no choice in the situation, many relatives will assume that you are in charge of everything and that you will call on them for help as needed.

Struggling to meet the demands of having too much to do and not enough time to do it can be eased by sharing the workload. Even out-of-town relatives can be of help if you will accept it. I understand there is the time element. Who has the time to teach another person the care you are providing? Isn't it easier just to keep doing it alone? It may seem that way, but I have seen over and over that when caregivers learn to share the burden, it provides a tremendous sense of relief.

Others probably won't do things the same way you will, but that's okay. You can train them on the important things, such as managing medications and safety. While it initially may feel like *more* work, it will be worth the time because eventually you will get a break. Training others to ease your load is a time investment, not a time cost. Of course, your loved one will likely have some misgivings about bringing other people into their routines, and that will need to be addressed in order to smooth the transition.

If you are a parent, you may recall what it felt like to try a new babysitter or to orient your child to a new daycare or school. You likely worried for them in a similar way: "Would everything work out okay?" But if you try to exude confidence that your loved one can handle it, they will pick up on it and be more likely to adjust. From my experience, if the transition is handled well, people can and do adapt.

You may need to start by arranging a family meeting or having a video conference to discuss your needs, everyone's availability, and even the option to seek help from outsiders. While dividing tasks among you may work well in the early days, as the demands grow, you may want to consider bringing in an aide or a care manager. It really can ease the stress that comes from handling things alone. Finding people to share the workload, even temporarily, will give you some time to relax and regroup.

Locating Help

When there is only one child in the family, the stress of caring for their aging parents or relatives can be immense. Some additional help is almost always needed. There are many sources of assistance, but it can take time to figure out exactly what you need. Your family member may have a trusted neighbor who is willing and has the time to help with some tasks, or you may need to hire one or more home care providers. Other options include senior centers, day programs for dementia patients, and other community resources. Many people are not aware that independent living residences and assisted living facilities offer what they call *respite care* opportunities to non-residents so that caregivers can get a much-needed break. You can read more about respite care in the appendix titled "Hiring Home Care Providers."

You can locate quality help for your loved one through internet research, word of mouth, local churches, or nonprofit organizations that coordinate volunteers to assist people in need. The appendix I mentioned details the types of home care providers available, explains how to utilize the services, and offers tips for introducing outside caregivers to your loved one. It also covers community programs and services for seniors, including low-income options.

If you don't figure out how to get a break, your body will eventually signal that you have taken on too much by hampering your immune system and decreasing your stamina. You may even become ill yourself. I have seen some stoic helpers who realized too late that help was needed. I want you to recognize it early so you can take care of yourself, too.

Whether or not you are able to get more help or temporary care, you will still need to take steps to reduce your stress on a regular basis in order to stay well and maintain the stamina necessary to fulfill your role.

Reducing Your Stress

Scientists have discovered in the last few decades that our physical brains—far from being "set" once we become adults—are actually quite adaptable. A simple change of perspective can, over time, literally change our brain structure. Just by changing how we think, we can help our brain become more resilient. A simple *gratitude practice* where we actively look for things to appreciate throughout the day can make a surprising difference in our attitude, as can healthy self-talk. Tell yourself "I am doing my best" as often as you need to hear it. Helping our brains work toward lessening our emotional burden isn't easy, and it takes time to form a new habit, but it can be done.

When we're stressed, our brains are wired to react in ways that aren't always best for the present situation. This can adversely affect our relationships. Researcher and author Jaqueline Brassey has coined the term *deliberate calm*, by which she means that you have a choice to be calm and intentional as you respond to any situation that you are facing. Her book *Deliberate Calm: How to Learn and Lead in a Volatile World* explains how to observe and recognize your typical style of responding, and then set an intention to change it. She encourages us to pay attention to what we're thinking and what we need, and says when we mess up, we should try to be gentle with ourselves.

Even small breaks from caregiving stress can make a big difference. If you're too overwhelmed to even think about reaching out for help right now, you can still help your body to relax by taking a moment here and there to focus on something calming in your environment. Tiny self-care habits like taking a moment for a deep breath can help our bodies calm down. We just don't always take the time to do them. Slow, calm, intentional breathing activates our body's natural relaxation response.

Many people are drawn to nature and find it soothing. Going outside for some sunshine feels good, but even viewing the natural world from your window can help. Look out the window to see birds and squirrels play or deer walk through your yard, depending on your locale. Just tracking the clouds as they pass by your window can relax you. Even a few moments of viewing nature can do wonders for you.

Try doing at least one thing each day that makes you happy, even if just for a few fleeting moments. Petting an animal, inhaling a gentle pleasant scent, having a laugh, or taking a nap can help you feel refreshed. Imagine that you are your best friend. What would he or she help you with now? Would they be gentle and kind with their words? You can become that kind to yourself too. Even though I often felt pushed for time, I started doing yoga and mindfulness meditation and found that I really enjoyed them. At one point, I also worked with a personal trainer to ensure that I had the physical strength to continue to do my job.

When we're stressed, we can easily lose our sense of humor, but levity can make life's challenges easier. When we laugh, it affects all kind of hormones in our bodies, increasing the positive ones and decreasing the negative ones. My dad had a great sense of humor, and he used to say he was "under new management" every time a different sibling came to town to assist him, which always made me chuckle. Sharing a laugh can help us bond with another person in the way few things can.

Speaking of bonding, make sure to take care of the social aspects of your life as well. You can have micro-connections with people just by texting for a few minutes or briefly chatting with someone you meet at a grocery store. Turn to supportive or funny friends who will brighten your day. Little positive moments throughout your day can be powerful mood elevators if you pay attention to them.

No matter the method, over time you can train your body to relax when you need it to, which will allow you to return to your work or family life a bit more refreshed.

After a break, when you do return to your loved one, be careful not to take any remaining stress back with you. I tell myself: "I will now put aside anything I am worried about or fearful about. I am going to be with my patient, and everything will be about them for a little while. I can get back to my own concerns when I take another break."

Finding Support

Individual therapy or counseling is another good option for stress relief. Since online therapy has become widely available, which makes scheduling simpler, more people have been motivated to give it a try to ease their uncomfortable feelings. Therapy can help you work through old family dynamics that may be increasing your frustration while caring for a parent or relative. The behavior of some seniors is so extreme that their caregivers may need support from a trained professional. These behaviors can often stem from unresolved childhood traumas or losses, and may have developed as coping mechanisms that loved ones have used for their whole lives.

Sharing what is going on by talking with someone who is eager to listen and asks the right questions is priceless. You can learn to deal more effectively with your own emotions, come to terms with your loved one's (especially a parent's) behavior and the likelihood that it will not change, and appropriately grieve losses of all kinds that you may be feeling.

The person you are caring for may even want to try therapy to give them some comfort and relief from their frustrations. Medicare pays for a large portion of in-home therapy services, although you may have to look around to find a provider that accepts Medicare. As your loved one's stress eases, it should make your job less difficult. I've mentioned how helpful therapy was to me throughout my life. It was truly a gift to me. What I learned there helped me to become happier, which helped my patients as well.

Support groups for caregivers are another good option. Many caregivers feel uncomfortable at first about joining a group. If you're highly independent, you may think you don't need or want to share. You may be surprised, though, to see how much *just talking* about your feelings and your needs may help. It can be especially helpful if you feel that other people really understand what you are going through. Finding out that you are not alone in your struggles sometimes makes them more bearable. You may even discover that your situation is actually not as difficult as someone else's. Although heartbreaking, it might alter your perspective a bit. Consider giving it a try—go to one meeting and see how you feel afterward. Take a friend with you if that would make you feel more comfortable. You may feel you don't have the time, but that one hour of support here or there might make all the difference in your overall attitude and energy level.

If you're not up for a meeting right now, you might try journaling what you are feeling on a regular basis. Looking back through your entries, you may notice some helpful trends, such as when your mood is starting to deteriorate, which indicates you should probably think about asking for more help or figuring out how to take a vacation if possible, or at least a break.

Our family members can help ease our burdens through simple acts of kindness to us if they know about our circumstances. Of course, you will have to share with them how you are feeling to some extent. One year while I was working on a Saturday, my teenage children surprised me by decorating the whole house for Christmas. It made me feel so relaxed and cared for.

Years later, I stopped by my grown daughter's new house and she could see that I was quite stressed due to my heavy schedule. She insisted that I take a few minutes to soak in her garden tub, and I could not believe how amazing it was! More recently, she has been calling me periodically to invite me to join her on her deck for a quick soak in her hot tub. It feels so good to be taken care of in those ways. It reminds us that our friends and family can provide some special treats to lift our mood if we allow them to. If you are a caregiver, you are a *helper*, and know the joy that can come from brightening someone else's day. Consider letting others feel a bit of that joy by helping *you* out from time to time.

Gradually the tide is turning, and we are finally beginning to understand that paying attention to our emotional health is essential to living a successful life. You may find that easing your stress will give you a whole new feeling about your current situation. This is your life too, and I sincerely want you to be happy.

Utilizing Other Resources

In the back of this book, you will find a Recommended Reading section, which has a list of many of the caregiving books I regularly reference. One I highly recommend is *Coping With Your Difficult Older Parent* by Barbara Kane. It has a terrific chapter on self-care that is well worth reading. In it, she says, "Do whatever works for you to release tension and to invigorate yourself so that your efforts will not drain you of energy and spirit."

In addition to books, there is a wealth of caregiver support resources including online support groups, websites, blogs, podcasts, social media sites, magazines, and newsletters. Here are a few of them:

Online support groups:
» Adult Children of Aging Parents: www.acapcommunity.org
   (for family caregivers)
» Aging Life Care Association: www.aginglifecare.org
   (for professional caregivers)

Websites:
» AARP Family Caregiving: www.aarp.org/caregiving
» Eldercare Locator: www.eldercare.acl.gov/Public/Index.aspx
» Aging Care: www.agingcare.com
» Caring.com resources for caregivers: www.caring.com/caregivers
» Caregiving.com resources for caregivers: www.caregiving.com
» Daily Caring: www.dailycaring.com
» Family Caregiver Alliance: www.caregiver.org
» Leeza's Care Connection: www.leezascareconnection.org
» Caring Today: www.caringtoday.com
» Tara Brach: www.tarabrach.com/caregivers
   (meditations for caregivers)

Podcasts/Blogs/Social Media Sites:

» The Best Podcasts for Family Caregivers: www.seniornavigator. org/article/78668/10-essential-podcasts-family-caregivers

» Top 90 Caregiver Blogs and Websites: www.blog.feedspot.com/ caregiver_blogs/

» 10 Favorite Caregivers on Instagram: www.thecaregiverspace.org/ our-10-favorite-caregivers-on-instagram/

Print and Digital Magazines:

» *Today's Caregiver* digital magazine: www.caregiver.com

» *Aging Well*: www.todaysgeriatricmedicine.com

» *Caregiver Solutions* digital magazine: www.caregiversolutions.ca

» *Chicago Health* caregiving magazine: www.chicagocaregiving. com

Here is a final story for you that illustrates the importance of allowing others to help:

She Gave Up All Her Free Time

One older couple I consulted with had a daughter, Amanda, who had moved in with them to help with their care. She became the primary caregiver for her parents, who had many needs. Her parents' care varied all the time, as one or the other became sick, had a fall, or were depressed. Amanda had many brothers and sisters. When I spoke with them, they all noted that Amanda was getting tired and so they had offered to help many, many times.

Amanda was single and thought she needed to be totally responsible for her parents since she had offered to live with them. She knew their needs so well that she felt it would take too much time and effort to teach the others. That feeling is completely understandable, yet can also lead to the possibility of burnout from constant caregiving. It was hard for Amanda to recognize that she was doing too much. She concentrated so much on her parents' care that she stopped having or even thinking about her own private life. She gave up all her free time to them. What a beautiful gift, except that her parents actually wanted her to have more freedom. They felt guilty about taking up so much of her time.

There was of course no easy answer to this situation other than to help Amanda recognize that she was tiring herself out. She needed to come to the realization that she was overdoing it and that the rest of the family *wanted* to participate in their parents' care as well. In situations like this, it's best to start changing things slowly. Maybe a sibling could start by doing the grocery shopping, cleaning the house, or offering to be with their parents a few hours every week to give Amanda some time off.

I reminded Amanda that the whole family wanted to be closer to her mom and dad, especially now, and that a loving thing she could do for her siblings and her parents was to *let the siblings participate* in some way. They did not want to take over her role and they didn't think they could do it better—they just wanted to be part of their parents' lives. It took some time for Amanda to really absorb this concept. Gradually, she was able to release a bit of her control and allow others to help, which eased the burden for everyone.

———————

The next time you're tempted to think that you would not be able to find or accept help, or that you don't have time for self-care, push back on that thought. If you find yourself becoming negative, this may be a warning sign that your own stress level is too high, and you need to increase your own self-care. You will need to figure out what works for your schedule and within your budget. Just trying out a few of the activities you learned in this chapter may brighten your spirits. I've talked with many family caregivers and I feel for your struggles. Keep trying new, creative ways to handle the stress of caregiving. You will be glad you did!

──────── **Key Takeaways** ────────

» The needs of aging seniors typically increase over time.

» Remember that your loved one's suffering is not your own. Taking on their suffering could impair your own energy.

» It is typical for caregivers to feel unappreciated by their family members.

» Chronic stress can lead to burnout, which can adversely affect both your health and your relationships.

» Directly involving siblings can enable them to be more realistic about what is possible.

» Ask for help rather than assuming others know what you need or that they will offer to help on their own.

» Find ways to recognize when you are not taking enough care of yourself.

» Think about what would give you relief from your current burden.

» Manage your stress and find some outlet for your feelings and needs, such as therapy.

» Pay close attention to your emotional health. It is essential for living a successful life.

──────── **Try It Out!** ────────

Think of one way you can be more compassionate
with yourself and start to implement it. Does it ease
your stress, brighten your mood, and help remind
you of the good you are doing in the world?

CONCLUSION

Most family caregivers really *want* to do a good job, but lack specific skills, especially when it comes to communicating effectively with their difficult loved ones. That's likely why you picked up this book—to learn some helpful tips.

I've spent a lifetime refining my skills and figuring out creative techniques and solutions that work to de-escalate rather than increase the tension between people. I don't expect you to be able to absorb them and use them right away just from reading through the book once. I hope I have shown you a new way to *think about* the many issues that can arise as you are caring for your family member.

Keep in mind that my suggestions are all aspirational—something to work toward. I know that on many days you *are* listening, being patient, and working hard to get along with your loved one as best you can.

I've tried my best to be encouraging and inspiring in these pages. Still, when you're struggling with an overwhelming task, it can be difficult to take in solutions from others. It can feel like they are "piling on" to your already heavy workload. I'm sensitive to that feeling. I've offered these tips for your consideration out of a genuine desire to *lessen* your load, and because I've seen them work time and time again. I'm confident that you can learn and apply them *in time*, as so many other family caregivers have, which will reduce your stress and help you to feel more successful.

Peaceful interactions contribute to the health and well-being of *both* the patient and the caregiver. Not only will learning how to react to your family member from a place of increased empathy make your job easier, but it will also make them happier and your relationship with them more satisfying. When you learn how to be more curious about, open to, and accepting of the needs of your aging parent or relative, it will carry over into all your relationships in the future. People *feel* it when we express genuine love and concern, and often they will reflect that back to us. I'm hoping the ideas you have learned from this book will help you say exactly what the world needs to hear in exactly the way it needs to be heard.

My goal was to offer you some tips to make your tough days a little easier, and to remind you to hang in there. Be gentle with yourself as you are learning these new techniques and testing them out. Caregiving is one of the most selfless acts of kindness we can offer to another person. I'm so proud of you for taking on this role, and I'm rooting for you!

———————

Thanks for reading. If you found this book helpful, please consider leaving an honest review on your favorite online bookstore's website.

HIRING HOME CARE PROVIDERS

As your family member ages, they may eventually need more help than you can provide. When this happens, your role may change from one of a direct, hands-on caregiver to a manager of trained home health aides or professionals. In this appendix I'll discuss when to bring in additional help, how to get your loved one and other family members on board, the various types of home care services available, how to hire and interact with staff, and the importance of having backup, no matter the level of care. I'll also address affordability and the availability of community resources for seniors.

Bringing in Home Health Care Providers

In Chapter 3, I talked about observing your loved one when you visit to assess any changes in their general health, hygiene, seeing and hearing, mood and demeanor, pain level, and the quality of their interactions with you and others. There are some signs that are clear indications that your family member may need more help than you're currently giving them—

perhaps they need weekly, twice weekly, daily, or even twenty-four-hour care. You may find that because their needs have increased, it's harder and harder to get out the door when you visit. If you see one or more of the concerning signs listed below, it may be time to speak with your loved one about their changing abilities and care needs.

Signs That May Indicate the Need for More or Specialized Help

» A sudden health event or diagnosis that requires more monitoring

» A deterioration significant enough that they can't perform the tasks they used to

» Complaints from your loved one that they "can't do all this" by themselves anymore

» Confusion to the point that they could harm themselves

» A sense that they would not be able to contact help if they needed it

» An indication from your family member that they are lonely

» A notification by one of their friends or neighbors that they are concerned about them (Remember the story of the Florida couple from Chapter 7?)

Preserving your own physical and mental health is an additional reason to bring in home health providers. This is especially important to be able to give your family member the best care you can offer them. You learned about emotional burnout in Chapter 12. The very best way to prevent it is to ask for help *before* you get to that point. Help can be hired also as a backup for you for the times when you are unavailable.

If you or other family members are unable to provide the next level of assistance, it's probably time to consider paying someone else to do it if the funds are available. There are different types of home health services and the decision about what type(s) to hire will depend on your loved one's unique situation. Sometimes more than one person, or more than one type of provider, is needed.

When you do decide to bring in additional help, on the one hand, you may be relieved to be getting some assistance with the daily tasks. On the other hand, coordinating care can still be time-consuming, and it may change the family dynamics a bit. It's all part of the journey.

Introducing the Idea of a Paid Caregiver

Caregiving often involves initiating difficult discussions, and one of the hardest is bringing up the idea that it may be time to hire outside help. As I have said before, there is no more important issue than your loved one's safety. Unfortunately, seniors often try to diminish the concerns of their adult children because they don't want to lose their independence. Try to broach the subject respectfully, and listen carefully to their concerns.

Many aging adults simply don't want strangers in their homes. This is probably the biggest hurdle to get over. You may have to ask them to simply "give it a try." Most seniors eventually learn to accept outside help and can even become quite attached to their paid caregivers.

The transition is the hard part, and your loved one will need your support to get through it. Often hiring occasional aides for light housekeeping and laundry works best, as they are most likely to want to give up those tasks. Consider starting this process before their needs become too great, and gradually increasing the level and frequency of care as needed. Be sure to be present during the first visit with each provider so the introduction goes smoothly.

Types of Home Care Services

In the health care field, there is a distinction made between professional providers and aides, who are not considered professionals. Professionals such as doctors, nurse practitioners, nurses, care managers, and therapists have much more extensive education and training and also must acquire and maintain a state license. Aides typically have six weeks of training and receive a certificate. They are required to have in-service training on fire safety, infection control, etc.

Home health agencies typically provide several different types of caregivers, depending on the need. The cost depends on the level of education and training the staff has. Each performs a specific type and level of care. Medicare pays for in-home assistance, both professional and aide services, for patients under certain circumstances if their doctor orders it. The patient must be confined to the home, and the doctor must deem the care medically necessary. A home health aide visit paid by Medicare can be up to two hours several times a week only when a skilled service like RN or PT are servicing as well. When the skilled service is discharged, Medicare no longer pays for the aide. See this government website for details: medicare.gov/coverage/home-health-services.

Your loved one's doctor will also be familiar with Medicare regulations and should be able to help you decide what kind of care your family member needs. You will want to familiarize yourself with these categories of helpers so you can make an informed choice after investigating your options:

Homemakers

While a patient is being medically cared for, a homemaker or person who helps with chores or tasks can maintain the household with meal preparation, laundry, grocery shopping, and other housekeeping items. Some also accompany patients to doctor visits, outings, or family events.

Home Care Companions

Companions spend time with your loved one and assist with activities. They do not provide medical care. Some provide transportation, accompanying people to doctor visits, outings, or family events.

Certified Nursing Assistants (CNAs)

Also called home care aides, these aides have taken coursework to be certified to better help the patient with daily personal needs such as getting out of bed, walking, bathing, and dressing. They often serve food, assist with activities, and help with exercise programs.

Certified Medication Aides (CMAs)

Some home care aides have received training to assist with more specialized care under the supervision of a nurse. They are permitted to dispense medications.

Professional Care Managers

Care managers are professional nurses or social workers or geriatric specialists who can replace you in your role of overseeing all aspects of your loved one's care, including managing the nurses and aides and communicating with all members of the team. These professionals are patient and family advocates, skilled at noting problems early and helping to proactively resolve them. They can provide guidance regarding living arrangements and help problem solve as issues arise. They can also help your loved one work toward increased safety, improved health, and fulfillment in life. Professional care management companies are paid privately unless your family member's long-term care insurance covers the service.

Medical Social Workers

Medical social workers provide various services, including counseling and locating community resources, to help patients in their recovery. Some social workers are also the patient's case manager, if the patient's medical condition is very complex and requires the coordination of many services.

Physical, Occupational, and Speech Therapists

Some patients may need help relearning how to perform daily duties or improving their speech after an illness or injury. A physical therapist can put together a plan of care to help a patient regain or strengthen use of muscles and joints. An occupational therapist can help a patient with physical, developmental, social, or emotional disabilities and help them relearn how to perform such daily functions as eating, bathing, dressing, and more. A speech therapist can help a patient with impaired speech to regain the ability to communicate clearly. All of these therapies are considered skilled services, which are provided under Medicare with a doctor's order, often upon release from the hospital after surgery or a medical event.

Registered Nurses (RNs) and Licensed Practical Nurses (LPNs)

The most common form of home health assistance is some type of nursing care, depending on the person's needs. In consultation with the doctor, a registered nurse will set up a plan of care. Nursing care may include wound dressing, ostomy care, intravenous therapy, administering medication, monitoring the general health of the patient, pain control, infection control, and other health support. Both types of nurses teach family members and other staff about any medical care that they may need to do. Registered nurses have the most training and can perform more medical procedures and treatments than licensed practical nurses, who provide similar care to RNs with a few limitations. Registered nurses oversee both licensed practical nurses and home care aides.

Physicians and Nurse Practitioners

Some doctors and NPs provide home-based care to chronically ill patients across age groups. They conduct assessments, diagnose disease conditions, order and provide treatment, and evaluate patient care. Doctors may also periodically review the home health care needs and write physician orders for a change of care. With the patient's permission, they are able to consult with family members for problems that might crop up.

Hiring Home Care Providers

Where to look: State and county Offices on Aging can be helpful by directing you to local community resources and programs. Most states/counties have prepared booklets listing all home care services. These booklets are available online, in libraries, in offices on aging, and in senior centers. Friends and neighbors may have names of services that have been helpful to them. The AARP website has a caregiving section with articles on all aspects of caregiving, including how to find and afford paid caregivers.

What to look for in an agency: Look for aide services that have a Medicare certification so they are able to contract with your professional services agency. (Medicare will not pay an aide to service on their own without an RN, PT, OT, social worker, or speech professional already being on the case.) Medicare agencies are surveyed annually by state staff based on a point system. You can investigate their Medicare survey scores on the Medicare website. Ask if an interview with the aide is provided. Also let the agency know about all other services that are currently servicing in your loved one's home. Ask about RN/LPN supervision of the staff.

What to look for in home health providers: No matter what level of provider you hire, look for people who have kind, calm, and happy demeanors, and who appear to be conscientious, good problem-solvers, and optimistic. If they enjoy what they do, it will show, and your loved one will respond positively to their good energy. Hopefully you will find people who display many of the traits I have talked about in this book.

How to explain your needs: When calling an individual or an agency to get help, be as specific as possible about your situation. Make a list before calling so you can give clear information about your loved one's needs. Will cooking be involved? Explain if transferring will be needed from bed to chair, which will require someone strong and experienced. Be sure to tell them about your loved one's personality, too. For example, let the agency representative know if your family member enjoys talking or prefers a quiet atmosphere, if they are timid or very directive or argumentative, and if they are a night owl or an early riser.

Working with professionals and aides: Communication is the most important factor when working with trained professionals. No matter who you contact, be sure to ask about availability and flexibility, the best ways and times to reach them, how and when they bill (including whether they are able to bill directly to long-term care insurance agencies if needed), and whether they provide backup personnel if they are unable to come. Once you have set up the service, the nurse or aide or therapist will contact you to arrange the individual appointments. If you need to change or cancel hours of service, let the agency know as soon as possible or there may be a charge. (A medical emergency is the exception.)

Documenting care: It can be helpful to have a notebook in the home with all of the personal information and emergency numbers that may be needed. Also, each provider should record the date and time of their visit and briefly note what they accomplished. Remember that they may not do things exactly as you would do them. Try to be flexible with them and allow them their own opportunities for creative problem solving.

Interacting with providers: Always be kind to all home care professionals and be clear about your expectations so that they will assist in a way that will satisfy your needs. When problems crop up, call the agency as soon as possible so that the issues can be resolved quickly. If the first person they send is not a good match, ask to try another. If you start off with honesty and good communication, working with professional staff and trained caregivers will be a successful and beneficial experience.

Private Agency Services Versus Private Non-Agency Services

The benefit of using an agency when you need a trained home care person is that the agency is responsible for employee supervision and for handling issues that crop up. The agency will bill you at intervals for the care. If your loved one has long-term care insurance, the bill may be sent to that company (who will then pay the agency) or it may be sent to you, depending on the arrangement.

Private home care people are often just as skilled as agency ones and may be less expensive, but there are some downsides to using them. The most challenging one is that most individuals do not have backups for themselves, so a family caregiver may have to step in at times. As their employer, you will have to provide oversight of the services they provide. Should they happen to get injured while working for you, or break something in the home, you will be responsible. You will also be responsible for HR functions such as hiring and firing help and making payments to them, including handling withholding taxes.

Always Have a Backup Plan for Care

Many family caregivers are reluctant to reach out for help because they feel they should be strong, or it's their job, but you can't be "on duty" twenty-four-seven. It's hard to break that mindset. It may not seem like there is anyone who can take your place, but there is. It's just a matter of finding them. What if you yourself were suddenly taken to the hospital— who would take over your caregiving role in that kind of emergency?

Finding a backup for yourself as soon as possible, even from the beginning of your caregiving role, is important. I am very aware that none of this is easy, and yet once you do it, you will find that it is so worth it for the peace of mind it will bring. Consider that there might be a neighbor or friend who is willing to help, but be sure to check with them ahead of time to see if they can be called upon in an emergency, or even for a few hours so you can occasionally regroup or take a refreshing walk.

When you do get to the point where you are able to hire home care providers, it's still important to have a backup plan to lessen your anxiety in the event there is an unexpected change. Paid caregivers can get sick or move, sometimes on short notice. Backup caregivers are especially important for family members who have dementia and can't be left alone even for a little while. If you have hired a care manager, that person can find the help you need for backup.

When You or Your Loved One Can't Afford to Hire Help

Many churches have programs to help aging adults, including providing financial support, housing assistance, home-delivery food service, and health care assistance. Call your house of worship to see if they have volunteers who can provide the help your loved one needs or can refer you to a national program like Catholic Charities, Jewish Family Services, or the Salvation Army for assistance.

Community Resources to Supplement Home Care

Respite care: As I mentioned in Chapter 12, some independent living residences and assisted living facilities offer non-residents what they call *respite care* opportunities so that caregivers can get a break. You can pay to have your loved one stay in an independent living residence for a few days or a week or two so you can go on vacation, attend an out-of-town family event, or take care of your own medical needs. Unfortunately, insurance does not cover these short-term stays, but the money you spend may be worth the reprieve you will get. The National Institute on Aging and AARP both have more information on respite care and how to find it in your area.

Respite care is a bit more complicated at assisted living facilities, but they do offer it. Usually, the person must be signed up for about a month. It requires a physician order as well as a medication and diagnosis list.

If you need to go out of town, respite can also be accomplished if another family member is willing to care for your loved one, either in their home or the family member's home. This allows another way for family caregivers to take a break. Communication and documentation are very important in these situations so the family members who are helping out know how to handle various scenarios that may arise.

Day Care: Your community likely offers day programs for seniors, which provide oversight and care to seniors for a half day or a full day. Lunch is provided and the fee is minimal compared to hiring a private aide. Day care provides socialization, which is so valuable to those who have little contact with others during the day. These programs are usually provided for seniors who need oversight and/or twenty-four-hour supervision, and they are a good way to supplement the care you are already providing. There are memory care day care centers that specialize in working with those with memory loss. And there are medical day care services, which are allowed to administer injections such as insulin. Transportation to and from the program is often provided within the local region.

Senior Centers: These drop-in centers offer programs and fun activities such as dance, music, and art for high-functioning seniors. Many even serve lunch. They often have exercise equipment, classes, and learning programs.

RECOMMENDED READING

Brackey, Jolene. *Creating Moments of Joy Along the Alzheimer's Journey: A Guide for Families and Caregivers.*
www.amazon.com/dp/1557537607

Brassey, Jacqueline. *Deliberate Calm: How to Learn and Lead in a Volatile World.*
www.amazon.com/dp/0063307642

Brown, Dr. Brené. *The Gifts of Imperfection.*
www.amazon.com/dp/1616499605

Brown, Steve. *How to Talk So People Will Listen.*
www.amazon.com/dp/0801016487

Hanson, Rick, PhD. *Making Great Relationships: Simple Practices for Solving Conflicts, Building Connection, and Fostering Love.*
www.amazon.com/dp/0593577930

Heath, Chip and Dan. *The Power of Moments: Why Certain Experiences Have Extraordinary Impact.*
www.amazon.com/dp/1501147765

Keirsey, David. *Please Understand Me II: Temperament, Character, Intelligence.* (Myers-Briggs Type Indicator)
www.amazon.com/dp/1885705026

Lebow, Grace and Barbara Kane. *Coping With Your Difficult Older Parent: A Guide for Stressed-Out Children.*
www.amazon.com/dp/038079750X

McDargh, Eileen. *Burnout to Breakthrough: Building Resilience to Refuel, Recharge, and Reclaim What Matters.*
www.amazon.com/dp/1523089466

Miller, R. and Stephen Rollnick. *Motivational Interviewing: Helping People Change.*
www.amazon.com/dp/1609182278

Noll, Douglas. *De-escalate: How to Calm an Angry Person in 90 Seconds or Less.*
www.amazon.com/dp/1582706557

Piemme, Laveta. *The Peaceful Eye of the Hurricane: Alternative Methods of Stress Relief for Caregivers.*
www.amazon.com/dp/B0981CQBPD

Rogers, Carl R. and Richard Evans Farson. *Active Listening.*
www.amazon.com/dp/1614278725

Rosengren, David B. *Building Motivational Interviewing Skills: A Practitioner Workbook.*
www.amazon.com/dp/1462532063

Solie, David. *How to Say it to Seniors: Closing the Communication Gap with our Elders.*
www.amazon.com/dp/0735203806

Sherts, Miles. *Conscious Communication: How to Establish Healthy Relationships and Resolve Conflict Peacefully while Maintaining Independence.*
www.amazon.com/dp/0985435917

Szalavitz, Maia. *Born For Love: Why Empathy is Essential—And Endangered.*
www.amazon.com/dp/0061656798

Todorov, Alexander. *Face Value: The Irresistible Influence of First Impressions.*
www.amazon.com/dp/0691167494

Turban, Melissa. *The Book of Boundaries: Set the Limits That Will Set You Free.*
www.amazon.com/dp/1785044400

ABOUT THE AUTHOR

Joan M. Foust, RN, has five decades of professional geriatric experience in hospitals, skilled nursing and rehab centers, and home health settings. As a geriatric care manager, her passion has been providing creative solutions to the unique challenges of senior living, particularly for patients with memory loss. She started HomeLife Services, LLC., to fill the gap in care when family members are unable to provide all of the support needed for their loved ones. She continues to share her knowledge through her writing and speaking engagements.

www.JoanMFoust.com
www.facebook.com/CreativeCaregivingSolutions

ACKNOWLEDGEMENTS

I am extremely thankful to have so many friends and family members and colleagues who supported me along my journey:

My dear husband Tim Foust was so supportive and patient during the whole process.

Special thanks to my sister Elaine Klonicki, a freelance writer, developmental and copy editor, and publisher. Her energetic work helped this book flow.

My son Drew Drozynski, Deputy Director of Business Development and Capacity Building at DevWorks International, grew up hearing my stories and then worked at HomeLife as a young adult. He contributed greatly to the writing and editing of the book, especially by calling me weekly in the early stage to help me get my narratives down and organized.

My daughter Kasia Sweeney, VP of Strategy at Calvert Health Medical Center, started HomeLife with me, then moved on to hospital management. Having worked in health care settings since she was teenager, she offered many insights about the needs of family caregivers.

My sister-in-law Emily Johnson was the initial one to suggest I write my patient stories down. Although it was not part of my life plan at the time, I slowly began to consider that my approach might be helpful for the tireless caregivers in the world.

My two good friends, nurse Mary Mitchell, and social worker Catherine LeMense, worked with me at HomeLife for many years and are quite proficient in using the methods offered in this book. They encouraged me to share them with other caregivers.

The following early readers were essential contributors, and their suggestions greatly enhanced the book:

My brother David Luddy, a caregiver himself, has been a powerful encourager.

My sister-in-law Sue Luddy, also a caregiver, was enthusiastic about the book's purpose.

My brother Steve Luddy called me weekly to provide encouragement and make me laugh.

My sister-in-law Debbie Luddy wrote beautiful emails that motivated me to continue writing. She was a careful reader, and her nonjudgmental honesty made the book better.

My sister Jeanie Silletti expressed much support and reminded me to encourage my readers to seek help early and often.

An extra shout-out to Myra McCrickard, PhD, who took the time to write an excellent analysis and provided some great ideas.

Mary Mitchell gave suggestions that led to the addition of the appendices.

Anna Bass has already started implementing my advice in the group she works with.

Diane Hay gave the book a thorough read and asked insightful questions which led to the addition of new material.

Several professionals assisted me during the creation of the book:

Lisa Hagan, a literary agent, read my book proposal and confirmed that my concept was a viable one.

Jenni Hart designed a draft of my front cover, offered sage advice throughout, and proofed the manuscript.

Zach Wiggin designed the book cover and interior and did the typesetting for it.

I am honored to have received beautiful endorsements from colleagues in many different fields:

Dr. Jean Fleming, former Executive Director of Calvert Hospice, who has a wealth of knowledge in the healthcare field.

Dr. Veena Alfred, an accomplished woman who owns multiple assisted living group homes, and runs them with great warmth and care. My clients were so happy in her homes.

Dr. Ted Tsangaris, a skilled surgeon whose warm bedside manner is noted by his patients. My respect for him is enormous.

Reverend Kirstin Tannas, pastor of Good Samaritan Lutheran Church, who inspires me with her sermons about kindness and compassion.

Lauren Simpson, a registered nurse and my former boss at Potomac Home Health. She guided me as I learned about the administrative end of healthcare services. I will forever be thankful that she chose me to be the Director of Professional Services.

Rick Amos, the leader of the Business Impact Group to which I belong. He greatly influenced my self-esteem by his appreciation for my ideas. He and the other members encouraged me to write my book, and finally I accepted the challenge.

Robert Bullock, Esq., owner of Elder & Disability Law Center. He is an enthusiastic and knowledgeable elder law attorney who sent many clients to HomeLife and called my staff "The Dream Team."

Nannette Vaughan, DNP, a nurse practitioner, educator, and national speaker about geriatric issues, provided helpful insights.

Barbara Kane, who owns a very successful care management company, was so kind as to agree to write the foreword. A pioneer in her field, as well as an author, Barbara made immense contributions to senior care. She inspired me to become a care manager, to start my own business, and to write this book.

Thank you all for taking the time to encourage my efforts, to read and offer suggestions, and to offer praise for the final version of the book.

INDEX

Made in the USA
Middletown, DE
16 October 2023

40872884R00126